SUCCESSFUL
PSYCHIATRIC PRACTICE

CURRENT DILEMMAS,
CHOICES, AND SOLUTIONS

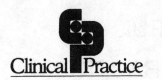

Clinical Practice

Number 33

Judith H. Gold, M.D., F.R.C.P.C.
Series Editor

SUCCESSFUL PSYCHIATRIC PRACTICE

CURRENT DILEMMAS, CHOICES, AND SOLUTIONS

Edited by

Edward K. Silberman, M.D.

Clinical Professor of Psychiatry
Thomas Jefferson University
Jefferson Medical College
Philadelphia, Pennsylvania

Washington, DC
London, England

Note: The authors have worked to ensure that all information in this book concerning drug dosages, schedules, and routes of administration is accurate as of the time of publication and consistent with standards set by the U.S. Food and Drug Administration and the general medical community. As medical research and practice advance, however, therapeutic standards may change. For this reason and because human and mechanical errors sometimes occur, we recommend that readers follow the advice of a physician who is directly involved in their care or the care of a member of their family.

Books published by the American Psychiatric Press, Inc., represent the views and opinions of the individual authors and do not necessarily represent the policies and opinions of the Press or the American Psychiatric Association.

Copyright © 1995 American Psychiatric Press, Inc.
ALL RIGHTS RESERVED
Manufactured in the United States of America on acid-free paper
First Edition   98   97   96   95   4   3   2   1

American Psychiatric Press, Inc.
1400 K Street, N.W., Washington, DC 20005

Library of Congress Cataloging-in-Publication Data
Successful psychiatric practice : current dilemmas,
   choices, and solutions / edited by Edward K. Silberman.
       p.   cm. — (Clinical practice ; #33)
   Includes bibliographical references and index.
   ISBN 0-88048-486-1 (hardcover : alk. paper)
     1. Psychiatry—Practice—United States.   2. Psychiatry—Practice—
United States—Case studies.   3. n-us.   I. Silberman, Edward K.,
1944- .   II. Series.
     [DNLM: 1. Psychiatry—trends.   2. Professional Practice—trends.
3. Psychotherapy—trends.   W1 CL 767J v. 33 1995 / WM 21 S942 1995]
RC465.6.S83   1995
616.89′0068—dc20
DNLM/DLC
for Library of Congress   95-1184
                                                                         CIP

British Library Cataloguing in Publication Data
A CIP record is available from the British Library.

Contents

Contributors

Richard K. Baer, M.D.
Associate Medical Director, Medicare of Illinois, Chicago, Illinois

Vicki Burnett, R.N.
Research Medical Center, Kansas City, Missouri

Judith H. W. Crossett, M.D., Ph.D.
Cedar Centre Psychiatric Group, Cedar Rapids, Iowa

R. Rao Gogineni, M.D.
Head of Ambulatory Care, Cooper Hospital Medical Center, Camden, New Jersey

Neil Goldman, M.D.
Private Practice, New York, New York

Leonard S. Goldstein, M.D.
Northern Virginia Psychiatric Group, Inc., Fairfax, Virginia

Dominic Mazza, M.D.
Private Practice, Scranton, Pennsylvania

Kathryn Ouzts, M.D.
Private Practice, Mt. Pleasant, South Carolina

Kenneth Piotrowski, M.D.
Private Practice, Sarasota, Florida

John D. Pro, M.D.
Midwest Psychiatric Consultants, Kansas City, Missouri

Harvey L. Rich, M.D.
Private Practice, Washington, DC

Boris Rifkin, M.D.
Private Practice, New Haven, Connecticut

Edward K. Silberman, M.D.
Clinical Professor of Psychiatry, Thomas Jefferson University,
Jefferson Medical College, Philadelphia, Pennsylvania

Otto H. Spoerl, M.D.
Group Health Cooperative of Puget Sound, Seattle, Washington

David van Dyke, M.D.
Private Practice, Viroqua, Wisconsin

Kenneth J. Weiss, M.D.
Medical Director, Delaware Valley Research Associates, King of
Prussia, Pennsylvania

Introduction

to the Clinical Practice Series

*O*ver the years of its existence the series of monographs entitled *Clinical Insights* gradually became focused on providing current, factual, and theoretical material of interest to the clinician working outside of a hospital setting. To reflect this orientation, the name of the Series has been changed to *Clinical Practice.*

The Clinical Practice Series will provide books that give the mental health clinician a practical, clinical approach to a variety of psychiatric problems. These books will provide up-to-date literature reviews and emphasize the most recent treatment methods. Thus, the publications in the Series will interest clinicians working both in psychiatry and in the other mental health professions.

Each year a number of books will be published dealing with all aspects of clinical practice. In addition, from time to time when appropriate, the publications may be revised and updated. Thus, the Series will provide quick access to relevant and important areas of psychiatric practice. Some books in the Series will be authored by a person considered to be an expert in that particular area; others will be edited by such an expert, who will also draw together other knowledgeable authors to produce a comprehensive overview of that topic.

This book discusses the various choices available for psychiatric practice today. The chapters consist of personal accounts by psychiatrists working in a variety of settings. Their experiences and comments will be valuable to those completing training and trying to make decisions about their future practice as well as to those psychiatrists who are considering changing their present mode of work. As such, this book adds to the earlier publications about private practice published by this Press.

Some of the books in the Clinical Practice Series will have their foundation in presentations at an annual meeting of the American Psychiatric Association. All will contain the most recently available information on the subjects discussed. Theoretical and scientific data will be applied to clinical situations, and case illustrations will be utilized in order to make the material even more relevant for the practitioner. Thus, the Clinical Practice Series should provide educational reading in a compact format especially designed for the mental health clinician–psychiatrist.

Judith H. Gold, M.D., F.R.C.P.C.
Series Editor
Clinical Practice Series

Clinical Practice Series Titles

Predictors of Treatment Response in Mood Disorders (#34)
Edited by Paul J. Goodnick, M.D.

Successful Psychiatric Practice: Current Dilemmas, Choices, and Solutions (#33)
Edited by Edward K. Silberman, M.D.

Alternatives to the Hospital for Acute Psychiatric Treatment (#32)
Edited by Richard Warner, M.B., D.P.M.

Behavioral Complications in Alzheimer's Disease (#31)
Edited by Brian A. Lawlor, M.D.

Clinician Safety (#30)
Edited by Burr Eichelman, M.D., Ph.D.

Effective Use of Group Therapy in Managed Care (#29)
Edited by K. Roy MacKenzie, M.D., F.R.C.P.C.

Rediscovering Childhood Trauma: Historical Casebook and Clinical Applications (#28)
Edited by Jean M. Goodwin, M.D., M.P.H.

Treatment of Adult Survivors of Incest (#27)
Edited by Patricia L. Paddison, M.D.

Madness and Loss of Motherhood: Sexuality, Reproduction, and Long-Term Mental Illness (#26)
Edited by Roberta J. Apfel, M.D., M.P.H., and Maryellen H. Handel, Ph.D.

Psychiatric Aspects of Symptom Management in Cancer Patients (#25)
Edited by William Breitbart, M.D., and Jimmie C. Holland, M.D.

Responding to Disaster: A Guide for Mental Health Professionals (#24)
Edited by Linda S. Austin, M.D.

Psychopharmacological Treatment Complications in the Elderly (#23)
Edited by Charles A. Shamoian, M.D., Ph.D.

Anxiety Disorders in Children and Adolescents (#22)
By Syed Arshad Husain, M.D., F.R.C.P.C., F.R.C.Psych., and Javad Kashani, M.D.

Suicide and Clinical Practice (#21)
Edited by Douglas Jacobs, M.D.

Preface

This book is about how successful practices of psychiatry are chosen, developed, and maintained. It is written at a time when increased oversight of mental health services and competition among providers have already brought considerable change in the climate of psychiatric practice, and more change is in the forecast. Psychiatrists, like others in times of change, may become preoccupied with bemoaning the loss of things as they used to be and scanning for signs of forthcoming disaster. However, despite changes in the conditions of practice, psychiatrists continue to thrive in a variety of practices in different settings.

The purpose of this book is to present first-person accounts by psychiatrists who have not merely survived, but who have maintained rich, rewarding practices in a period of change and uncertainty. Rather than report statistical data on trends in practice, we have chosen to relate the personal experiences of psychiatrists who have struggled and dealt successfully with the changes currently taking place in psychiatric practice. Although the authors of these chapters represent a sample intentionally skewed in the direction of success, they are typical of private practioners in the way they have focused and developed their careers. The means to success they describe are available to anyone with clearly defined goals and the will to work toward them consistently over time.

The first chapter presents an overview of forces that are currently shaping psychiatric practice and the ways in which modes of treatment and styles of practice have been changing. The chapters that follow describe a variety of practice types in diverse settings: solo, group, and institutional practice; urban, small-city, and rural practice; and general and subspecialty practice. Chapters are also included on practice in a staff-model health maintenance organization (HMO), a new and growing form of practice in the private sector, and on practice as a salaried hospital staff member. The latter may be a full-time form of practice in itself or may also be a part-time supplement to office-based practice. The authors describe the goals and interests that led them to their type of practice, the development of the practice, its distinctive features, and how they have maintained it in the face of economic pressures, competition, and managed care. They discuss the training necessary for their work, their relationships with colleagues and competitors, the compromises they have had to make, their false starts and mistakes, and the rewards of practicing how and where they do. We hope that the experiences of the authors will be useful to those starting their careers and that the practices they describe will be relevant models for the present and future.

Edward K. Silberman, M.D.

Chapter 1

Changes and Dilemmas in Psychiatric Practice

Boris Rifkin, M.D.

*D*uring the past 15 years, dramatic changes have occurred in the field of psychiatry, which have affected every aspect of private practice. The changes have been driven by several factors, including the need to decrease costs, advances in psychiatric treatment, the role of nonpsychiatric therapists, and legal and legislative issues. In this chapter, I summarize these factors and what effect they have had on income, style and structure of practice, administrative work, and levels of satisfaction.

Changes in Psychiatric Treatment

During World War II, psychiatric care became synonymous with psychoanalysis, and in those cases in which a less intense approach was indicated, insight-oriented psychotherapy. This resulted when psychoanalysts from Europe came to the United States and offered the first viable treatment approach. Over the years other treatments were developed in response to dissatisfaction with the outcome of psychoanalytic therapy and the need for briefer therapy to treat the increased numbers of patients seeking psychiatric care. This need coincided with the development of other theories and consequent new and different techniques. The best known and most influential of these approaches have been brief therapy developed by Sifneos (1979) and Davanloo (1978), behavior therapy developed by Wolpe and Lazarus (1966), cognitive therapy by Beck et al. (1979), and interpersonal therapy by Weissman and co-workers (1981). Coincident with changes in the type of psychotherapy was change in the format of therapy;

techniques such as group therapy and family therapy grew rapidly.

Another important development was the advent of psychopharmacology as a significant treatment approach. Antidepressants and phenothiazines shortened the treatment period and allowed many hospitalized patients to be discharged. Furthermore, the development of partial hospital and crisis intervention programs lessened the use of increasingly expensive hospitals.

Funding sources used all of these changes in the approach to treatment to reduce the cost of psychiatric care. State and federal funding sources, along with insurers and managed care companies, strongly encouraged these new approaches to shorten both inpatient and outpatient treatment and, in many cases, to prevent hospitalization. Some authorities began to predict that by the year 2000 psychotherapy would be much more focally targeted and more cognitively and behaviorally oriented (Sabshin 1993).

Competition With Other Professionals

As the need for psychiatric treatment expanded, psychiatrists began to train different, but related, disciplines to assist with their work. This engagement began with psychology and social work. Psychology had begun as a separate discipline that concentrated on research and psychological testing and gradually moved into the area of therapy. Approaches within clinical psychology ranged from psychoanalysis to behavior therapy. Training was extensive and consisted of a Ph.D. and an internship, but no experience in medical or pharmacological fields. Social workers were the next discipline to be incorporated into assisting with therapy. Their origins dated back to the influence of Adolph Meyer (1957) at the turn of the century. Initially, this field concentrated on social and family issues. More recently, therapy has begun to be provided by nurse practitioners with master's degrees in psychiatric nursing and a variety of other disciplines with varied skills. These include master's-level psychologists, pastoral counselors, nurses, and psychiatric technicians, usually with 2-year degrees.

Over the years, these groups began to develop their own professional organizations and became active in private practice and politics. The first and most active group was the psychologists; they have achieved significant changes to date through both legislative and legal action. These changes include licensure in many states and, thus, the ability to collect third-party payments for private practice, the right to admit to hospitals (in California), and the development of a trial program of prescription writing by psychologists in the military. Efforts by nonmedical professional organizations continue to expand hospital admission privileges and psychologist prescribing practices to other areas and also lead to new domains such as ability to institute commitment. Other groups have attempted to obtain licensure with variable results. Social workers and nurse practitioners are recognized by most states, but other groups have had far less success. Nurse practitioners have also been approved for prescribing psychotropic drugs in many states with little opposition, probably because their training is far more medically oriented than that of psychologists. Primary care physicians, internists, and pediatricians also interact with psychiatrists in some areas. This group sees many patients before they are referred to psychiatrists and often prescribes psychotropic drugs. They sometimes work together with other therapists, such as psychologists or social workers, to provide a therapeutic program for patients who need mental health services.

Difficulties With Reimbursement

The earliest form of reimbursement for psychiatric care was direct payment by the patient to the psychiatrist. Gradually, as psychiatric care expanded, the need for broader financial backing grew. This need was driven by factors such as hospitalization and the necessity to provide care for patients who required financial assistance. In this section, I describe the current major systems of reimbursement.

Indemnity Insurance

The first form of third-party coverage for psychiatric care was indemnity insurance, usually provided by a major medical policy. Initially, the costs were not significant because of low patient utilization and the low cost of hospital care, and coverage was frequently 80%. Gradually, costs rose as a result of increased use of long-term hospitalization, particularly for adolescents. The third-party payers were quite concerned because overall medical costs were rising at a much higher rate than the cost of living. They believed that psychiatric care was not as essential as general medical care and that state hospitals were available to treat the more disturbed patients. Therefore, insurance companies began to persuade employers to decrease their psychiatric coverage and devised several alternatives to achieve this goal. These consisted of reducing the payment of benefits from 80% to 50% and applying caps to the total amount of money payable for psychiatric care. State psychiatric societies responded by encouraging legislators to mandate minimum benefits and were successful in some cases. More recently, the advent of managed care, along with the development of health maintenance organizations (HMOs) and preferred provider organizations (PPOs), have served to significantly reduce psychiatric benefits.

HMOs

HMOs were developed to reduce health care costs. The federal government offered financial and other means of support for their development and was prepared to use legal and legislative means to discourage any organized opposition. HMOs are divided into two models—a closed service type and an Independent Practice Association (IPA) model. The closed service model is staffed by salaried physicians, mostly full time, and is of little interest to private practitioners other than as a part-time salaried position. In the IPA model, an insurance company or other developer negotiates with a group of physicians to provide medical services to their patient population (American Psychiatric Association 1985). The IPA negotiates on behalf of the physicians. Negotiations include setting fees, reviewing and altering contracts, and performing utilization review and peer review. The negotiations can be complex, and it is important for the physicians who handle the negotiations to have a good understanding of contracts and antitrust laws. From the psychiatric point of view, there is the usual difference between medical and psychiatric benefits. Fees tend to vary from reasonable and equitable to minimum, and outpatient treatments range from 6 visits to as high as 30. Inpatient treatments are also subject to caps on the length of stay. The advantages of the IPA system is that physicians are protected by the IPA, which has the power to negotiate on their behalf. HMOs are often developed and limited to hospital staffs, in which the same principles and systems apply, and are then called hospital practice organizations (HPOs).

PPOs

PPOs are somewhat similar to HMOs, but there are some distinct differences. PPOs are developed by an insurance company or other health funding agency. In contrast to HMOs, no negotiation body (such as an IPA) represents the physicians. In fact, because of current antitrust laws, it is risky to speak to other physicians about fees or the advisability of joining. PPOs are offered to physicians with a definitive contract and a fixed fee schedule, with no possibility of changing or renegotiating them. The fees are usually lower than those allowed by indemnity insurance contracts, and limits are often set on the amount of inpatient and outpatient treatment allowed. Because of the paucity of physician advice for PPO participation, psychiatrists who are not familiar with contracts should consult an attorney, a medical society, or a psychiatric society before signing a PPO contract. I explain some of the risks and pitfalls of these contracts in the section, "Legal and Related Issues."

Managed Care

Managed care is a procedure to evaluate medical treatment by monitoring its efficiency, effectiveness, and quality. Procedures can be designed for both the public and the private sectors, but often its application to the private sector is mainly focused on reducing cost. The managed care approach is being used for this purpose by all the funding sources, including indemnity insurers, HMOs, and PPOs. Managed care is provided by organizations that are separate from the funding sources, and it is usually applied to all branches of medicine. However, in many cases a separate source provides the managed care for psychiatry. In the psychiatric section, managed care is often based on review of the necessity for treatment (Rifkin 1991). All health care funding sources stipulate a maximum number of inpatient days and outpatient visits in their contracts. However, managed care reviewers do not always grant the maximum benefit. Reviewers now demand a preadmission screening before they agree to admission, and they do not agree to admit in every case. Furthermore, once the patient is admitted, they insist on reviews every 2 to 7 days, and they demand additional justification for extending the length of stay.

Outpatient care has also recently come under regular review. Some companies review outpatient treatment at fixed-interval visits, usually ranging from five to ten, before they agree to further treatment. Other companies evaluate the patient with the psychiatrist following the intake and then decide on the frequency and number of visits allowed before the next review. When the company reviews patients, the psychiatrist is obligated to provide a 10- to 20-minute telephone interview for each review, with no reimbursement. The effect of managed care has been to dramatically shorten the length of stay in psychiatric inpatient settings. In many cases the number of empty inpatient beds has increased markedly, and hospital wards and private psychiatric hospitals are being closed down. The most recent intervention by managed care companies is to reduce admission further by vigorous use of day hospitals and to financially support intensive outpatient care, because the cost of 1 day in a general hospital can be as high as the cost of ten outpatient visits. The number of outpatient visits per patient illness is also decreasing, as psychiatrists feel pressure to justify their treatment in the face of persistent outpatient review. In their efforts to further reduce costs, some independent reviewers tend to suggest treatment approaches, such as cognitive therapy or antidepressants, and, in some cases, insist on treatment with social workers, claiming that their evaluation and treatment are better, and they charge less.

Legal and Related Issues

Contracts

Prior to the advent of HMOs, psychiatrists never worried about contracts unless they were entering into a partnership, a lease, or a similar business-related venture. However, now most psychiatrists sign several contracts each year, often, unfortunately, without reading or understanding them. Currently, the majority of these contracts are related to HMOs and PPOs, and the following areas should be identified and evaluated by psychiatrists before signing.

* *Fees and limits on treatment:* For an HMO, the IPA negotiates fee packages on behalf of its members. The fees offered by a PPO are set by the funding agency. According to antitrust laws, physicians cannot discuss fees or bargain as a group with funding agencies. The IPA

can negotiate fees, but the only physician input permitted is a survey by the IPA of usual and customary fees. The results of the survey should not be shared with the membership. The psychiatrist must then decide on his or her own whether the fee is acceptable and, thus, whether to join. In addition to fees, it is important to note what type of treatment package is offered. If, for example, the contract offers 6 outpatient visits and 7 inpatient days, each psychiatrist must decide whether he or she is comfortable providing treatment within these limits and whether to participate. Again, negotiation is only permitted by the IPA.

* *Hold harmless clauses and peer review:* Many contracts include a hold harmless clause. This is a statement that if any legal action is taken against the company for whatever reason, the psychiatrist agrees to hold the company harmless and, thus, exposes himself or herself to all the legal risk. Note that nearly all malpractice policies, including the American Psychiatric Association–sponsored group, state in their contracts that if psychiatrists sign a hold harmless clause, it is a breach of contract, and they will not be covered by their own insurer. Therefore, a hold harmless clause should never be signed because it voids an individual's malpractice policy (American Psychiatric Association 1992). HMOs may also require psychiatrists to take part in peer review, and many malpractice policies deny coverage for suits arising out of peer review. Some policies, including the American Psychiatric Association, do provide coverage in this area. However, even if you do have coverage, peer review participation should still be thought out very carefully; although participation is a worthwhile endeavor, suits arising out of this area are often of the antitrust variety in which the concept of insurance coverage is unclear and confusing.

* *Referrals and gatekeepers:* Both HMO and PPO contracts sometimes allow patients to go directly to psychiatrists by reading their names in the published list of accepted treating physicians. Patients might also be directly referred by their physician or, in rarer instances, by work sources, such as an Employee Assistance Program (EAP), or by the insurer itself. Most psychiatrists prefer this type of contract, and it generally presents no problems. Many contracts, however, use a gatekeeper system. Most gatekeepers are primary care physicians. In this type of system, the psychiatrist should have relationships with a number of referral sources or develop such relationships in order to make joining the program worthwhile. Some primary physicians prefer

to refer the majority of their psychiatric patients, but others attempt to treat as many of their own patients as possible. More difficulties might arise when the gatekeepers are paid a bonus for treating these cases themselves. Another gatekeeper that might give psychiatrists problems is the social worker or psychologist. In this model, most cases requiring therapy will be referred to nonmedical therapists. The psychiatrist's role is to medicate patients and provide an occasional backup consultation.

* *Issues of payment:*   Payment for patients in HMOs and PPOs is made directly to the psychiatrists, except for a copayment by the patient that varies from program to program, but is usually less than 50%. The amount of payment and the eligibility for treatment are spelled out in the contract. The advantage of these plans is that a large part of the fee is paid directly to the psychiatrist. However, some difficulties may arise. First, many HMOs have a withhold, which means that a certain portion of the fee, usually 20%, is kept back and only paid if the HMO makes a profit. In our experience, in most cases the withheld money is not returned because most programs seem to run at a loss (Rifkin 1987). One further complication is that certain contracts state that if there is a severe negative cash flow, the withhold can be increased to 30% or more to make up for the loss; this is described as part of the physician risk sharing.

  A second way of dealing with HMO shortfalls is to provide the IPA with a fixed amount per case and to hold the physicians responsible for any deficit, including hospital costs. This arrangement might have considerable risk for the psychiatrist. HMO and PPO contracts usually last for a year; renewal is an option for both parties, so psychiatrists may find that their contract has unilaterally not been renewed by the HMO. In addition, if the program runs out of funds and declares bankruptcy, the psychiatrist is obligated to treat the patient without remuneration until the contract ends or an acceptable alternative treatment is found. Contracts should state that interest will be payable to the psychiatrist when payment is more than 30 days late.

When considering joining an HMO or PPO, it is important to review the contract and, if some of the above negative points exist, to attempt to have them changed through the IPA. If that route is not possible, these factors may outweigh the benefits of joining the program.

Antitrust

Antitrust issues were unheard of in the field of medicine a few years ago, but in recent years, they have become infrequent, but very significant. Antitrust risks for the private practitioner occur mainly in the area of HMOs, PPOs, and hospital staff privileges. The particular offense, closely watched for by the Federal Communications Commission, is any attempt to discuss and thereby influence fee schedules. Furthermore, any attempt to discourage physicians from joining these organizations, either in writing or through verbal communications, is very dangerous. The penalties for antitrust are both civil (usually triple charges) and criminal and usually are not covered by insurance. Therefore, psychiatrists must be extremely careful when dealing with HMOs and PPOs that they do not discuss fees or act in any way that might publicly discourage other physicians from joining the programs. Another area in which antitrust has become a factor is that, if, as a consequence of peer review, a physician is denied or loses hospital or HMO privileges, that physician may sue the members of the committee under federal antitrust laws. These suits cannot be prevented by state exemptions for antitrust for hospital peer review committees. Finally, it is important to keep antitrust in mind with the new interest in the development of groups of physicians or therapists who can be negotiated with under the managed competition model. Doctors left out of such groups might consider suing on an antitrust basis. Therefore, legal consultation in setting up these groups is essential to protect the physician.

Malpractice

Practicing psychiatrists should be knowledgeable about the types and limitations of malpractice policies. There are two main types of policies—occurrence and claims made. Occurrence is difficult to find today, but it is offered by the American Psychiatric Association–sponsored company. With this type of policy, all incidents that occur while the policy is in force are covered, regardless of how many years after the incident the suit is filed. In the claims-made variety, coverage is only active while the policy is in force, and physicians who leave the program must take out a "tail policy" to cover future claims. Such policies are often very expensive. In some cases, a modified tail is available as the physician reaches retirement age. Most hospitals and HMOs require a minimum of $1 million of malpractice coverage.

The two cornerstones of prevention in malpractice are record keeping and second opinions. Records should be precise, spell out the reasons for all the actions taken, and record the medication used and details of the side effects. Special evaluations, such as use of the Abnormal Involuntary Movements Scale (AIMS) for tardive dyskinesia or pulse and blood pressure, should be recorded. Above all, records should never be altered at a later date, but a note can be added if the entry is clearly dated. A second opinion is always valuable whenever there is any doubt about the treatment, diagnosis, or management. The filing of malpractice suits and the dollar amount of awards have been increasing; in rare cases, they have exceeded the American Psychiatric Association's $1 million coverage limits. Today's practice is extremely complicated, and a malpractice suit can be brought against a psychiatrist for a variety of reasons. However, if one practices good medicine and keeps the above guidelines in mind, malpractice should not be a major problem.

Ethics and Fraud

The main ethical concern for private practitioners is a relationship with a patient that breaches boundaries, especially those that lead to sexual involvement. The nature of these infringements is well noted in *The Principles of Medical Ethics With Annotations Especially Applicable to Psychiatry,* the details of which are readily accessible to psychiatrists (American Psychiatric Association 1993). Practitioners, however, should be aware that these regulations produce some extra risk for them and, therefore, might necessitate some changes in practice. First, private practitioners tend to work alone, without a secretary or another person sharing the office. This structure was selected because of finances and a desire to enhance privacy for the patient. However, in today's environment it is important to have someone in the office as much as possible. A secretary would provide the presence of another person in the office as well as valuable help with billing, making appointments, and handling messages. Another way to increase a presence in the office is to share space with other therapists, which helps to create a less private and intimate atmosphere. Furthermore, psychiatrists who use different approaches, such as behavior therapy, are faced with a significant problem, because such techniques might be seen as violating boundaries. The American Psychiatric Association must closely examine these alternative techniques in order to develop specific guidelines for them.

Apart from obvious fraud, such as billing for treatment that was not provided, several other business-related behaviors might be regarded as ethical violations. First, it is expected that there will be one standard fee for each procedure, and if a patient receives a reduced fee, the rationale should be well documented. The reason for this is that insurers believe that some psychiatrists might bill them a high fee and then, once the insurer pays, reduce the copayment for the patient. Another problematic area is attempting to bill insurers for missed appointments, which are not covered by most insurance plans. In certain cases the patient may be billed, but this arrangement should be clearly spelled out at the beginning of treatment. Also, bills covering telephone calls and work done by nonpsychiatric therapists should clearly indicate the procedure and who has provided the service. Finally, psychiatrists should not use information obtained from patients during therapy sessions for financial gain, such as investing in the stock market.

Current and Future Trends in Private Practice

Although the changes in private practice of psychiatry have been considerable over the last 10 to 15 years, the degree to which practitioners are affected varies greatly. Psychiatric practice in California, for example, has been shaped by managed care much more than in New York. However, the trend clearly is toward greater third-party oversight and restrictions in treatment and fees in all geographic areas. These trends, plus the increasing burden of time spent documenting treatment and negotiating with payers, are the major causes of demoralization among practitioners.

The nature of psychiatric practice has begun to change in response to economic, regulatory, legal, and competitive pressures. An American Psychiatric Association survey in 1986 showed that full-time solo private practice was the mode for less than one-half of active psychiatrists, and the decline has continued. Instead, more psychiatrists are practicing in groups or as part of managed care organizations, such as HMOs. More time is being spent in brief psychotherapy or medication management; less time is being spent in long-term outpatient therapy, and drastically less time in management of long-term inpatient treatment.

Also note, however, that the same American Psychiatric Association survey showed that a vast majority of psychiatrists still spend *some* portion of their professional time as solo private practitioners. Whether this will continue to be the case depends to some degree on the type of national health care system that is put into place. However, the current message is that for most psychiatrists, the core of clinical practice, but not the range, has shifted considerably. At present, then, there is room for a great variety of practice types, although there is far less autonomy for psychiatrists than was once the case.

Whatever the future holds, psychiatrists will best be able to maintain a meaningful role in health care by being proactive on their own behalf as well as flexible in adapting to change. Such activity means, among other things

• Becoming more involved with other physicians and emphasizing their medical role in mental health care
• Playing a leadership role on multidisciplinary teams
• Developing practice guidelines that help to define necessity and parameters of psychiatric treatment
• Learning and using brief forms of psychotherapy
• Becoming more politically active in influencing the legislative process

In these ways, psychiatrists will take part in shaping the future and maintaining a role in health care delivery.

References

American Psychiatric Association: An Economic Survival Manual for Private Practice Psychiatrists. Edited by Muszynski IL Jr. Washington, DC, American Psychiatric Press, 1985, p 23

American Psychiatric Association: Utilization Management: A Handbook for Psychiatrists. Washington, DC, American Psychiatric Association, 1992

American Psychiatric Association: The Principles of Medical Ethics: With Annotations Especially Applicable to Psychiatry. Washington, DC, American Psychiatric Association, 1993

Beck AT, Rush AJ, Shaw BF, et al: Cognitive Therapy of Depression. New York, Guilford, 1979

Davanloo H (ed): Basic Principles and Techniques in Short Term Dynamic Psychotherapy. New York, Spectrum, 1978

Meyer A (ed): Psychobiology: A Science of Man. Springfield, IL, Charles C Thomas, 1957

Rifkin BG: How to avoid the pitfalls of signing with managed care systems. Psychiatric News, November 6, 1987, p 17

Rifkin BG: Managed care and private practice in the 1990s. Psychiatric News, May 17, 1991

Sabshin M: Will psychiatrists provide psychotherapy in the year 2000? The Gap Reporter, November 1993, p 5

Sifneos P (ed): Short Term Psychotherapy Evaluation and Technique. New York, Plenum, 1979

Weissman MM, Klerman GL, Prussoff BA, et al: Depressed outpatients: results one year after treatment with drugs, and/or interpersonal psychotherapy. Arch Gen Psychiatry 38:51–55, 1981

Wolpe J, Lazarus AA (eds): Behavior Therapy Techniques. New York, Pergamon, 1966

Chapter 2

Urban Psychiatric Practice

Richard K. Baer, M.D.

*T*he large majority of psychiatrists in the United States practice in an urban setting. This may be because American psychiatrists are a particularly urbane lot. However, I think a more likely explanation is that psychiatrists, perhaps more than any other specialty, practice where they train. This is unfortunate for those areas underserved by psychiatrists, but understandable historically considering the nature of urban psychiatric practice.

Urban psychiatric practice has been chiefly office-based solo practice. Although most psychiatrists practice in more than one setting, office-based clinical practice has been the most common. In a national study, Dorwart and co-workers (1992) found that, in 1988, psychiatrists had a mean of 2.3 practice settings; 45.1% reported the office as their primary activity, and 25.8% reported the office as their most important secondary activity. In years past, the majority of psychiatric residents training in urban medical centers were expected to complete training and establish a private office practice. It was also the main interest of many psychiatric residency supervisors and other role models.

A Career Vision: Private Practice 30 Years Ago

During the 1960s and 1970s, psychoanalysis was the preeminent theory for understanding patients, and most psychiatric residency department chairmen and residency supervisors were analysts. This trend began to shift in the 1970s, and throughout the 1980s, a progressively more biological orientation predominated.

As this biological approach to understanding patients has increased, office-based practice has diminished. Office-based practice as a primary work setting decreased from 57.7% in 1982 (when I completed my residency training) to 45.1% in 1988 (Dorwart et al. 1992). I suspect this percentage has continued to decline into the 1990s as more psychiatrists become employed by large group practices, health maintenance organizations (HMOs), and other forms of corporate practice.

When I completed residency training in 1982 from a large midwestern state university urban medical center, managed care was only a gleam in the eye of an insurance executive. My psychoanalyst supervisors were flourishing in fee-for-service office-based practice, and full case loads of psychoanalytic patients were not rare among the city's leading psychoanalysts. This is how I saw myself living my professional life. Among residents there was a rumor that after graduating from certain training programs, the faculty would refer patients to you, and you would essentially be set up in practice. This rumor turned out to be about 10 years old; I spoke to one supervisor 20 years my senior whose case load was full of scheduled appointments weeks before the end of his residency, including patients seeking psychoanalysis.

Third-party reimbursement for outpatient psychotherapy was already decreasing in 1982. In 1980, I received my residency stipend from a veterans hospital, which provided federal insurance benefits. During that year, my insurance paid for 80% of my training analysis. In 1981, that was reduced to 70%, and more rapid cuts were soon to follow.

The vision of what I hoped and expected my practice to be was based on my supervisors' practices. My psychoanalytic-oriented supervisors primarily saw patients in their offices for treatment with psychotherapy or a combination of medication management and psychotherapy. They may have had a small hospital practice as well. Their practices were busy. They had a university affiliation, which gave them an opportunity to teach and have collegial relationships. They did volunteer work for their respective professional societies. Their expertise and experience grew with seeing patients year after year. This continued until the psychiatrist died; it was a way of life.

Encountering Reality

There was no preparation from my residency program for professional development post residency training. I simply assumed that developing an outpatient office practice in 1982 would be a little more difficult than it had been. I rented office space, bought some furniture, sent out hundreds of announcements, and began to see the few patients that were from my caseload as a resident.

Because I trained at a state university, I could not use that affiliation for hospitalizing private patients. I applied for and received admitting privileges at a small private psychiatric hospital where I knew no one. After 6 months, my practice was about one-half full, and I felt very isolated.

There were too many psychiatrists in the city. I also had no idea how to position myself on a career path toward the vision articulated above, and my situation in the winter of 1983 demonstrated that.

Establishing a Private Practice

Choice of Residency Training

Because I had intended to go into private practice, a residency program in a private university medical school, with a better model for private practice, would have better prepared me. It would have introduced me firsthand to psychiatrists who were practicing as I intended, and I could have continued my affiliation with the hospital, enabling me to admit my private patients. My supervisors and role models would have been more relevant to my ambitions, and I might have been able to enter into a partnership with one of them. In any case, the transition from training to practice would have been smoother.

Salaried Positions

Another solution would have been to take one of the many available part-time jobs following residency training. In Chicago, where I practice, there are six university medical schools and at least a dozen associated teaching hospitals outside the university campuses, all of which employ unit directors to administrate the teaching activities on the inpatient unit and to monitor the quality of patient care. In the university settings, the unit chiefs also have research work, teaching responsibilities, and medical school and residency administration work. Other full- or part-time entry-level positions also may exist in university settings. Outpatient services, consultation-liaison services, or other subspecialty services may have positions available in large university medical schools. These will vary between schools. Research done or papers published during residency may especially qualify a graduating resident for such a university position.

Private, nonteaching hospitals may offer a good salary or other benefits (such as secretarial services or office space) to psychiatrists who manage administrative responsibilities for the hospital. These positions should be sought only at the hospitals in which you hope to develop a practice. They will allow you to become intimately involved with the functioning and administration of the hospital, and your practice activities will become organized around that affiliation.

Public and private mental health centers employ psychiatrists for medication management, diagnostic evaluation, and administrative supervision of other mental health workers. There are dozens of these clinics in large urban centers. They require the psychiatrist to be a member of a multidisciplinary team of other psychiatrists, psychologists, social workers, and others.

The most common position available to residents as they complete training has been unit director on an inpatient psychiatric unit. It is either a quarter- or half-time position that serves several purposes. First, it provides an income on which to live and support office overhead while developing a private practice. Second, it involves you in the life of the hospital, and your daily presence is an opportunity to meet other doctors and develop sources of referral from physicians in other specialties. Third, this position may develop into other positions at higher levels of administrative responsibility in the department, or you may leave it as your private practice grows, opening it up for the next resident.

Today, the positions that are available to graduating residents are changing. Many HMOs that employ their own psychiatrists select residents coming out of training because they command a lower salary than someone who has been practicing for a while. As more medicine is practiced in large group or corporate settings, it will become more common to "take a job" with a group practice or HMO that consists almost exclusively of psychotropic medication management. Insurance companies and managed care entities are becoming employers of a number of psychiatrists as well; this could develop into a whole new career path.

Therapeutic Skills

As I learned, private practice is an entrepreneurial undertaking. Traditionally, the financial rewards have been greater in private practice, but so have the risks. Supply and demand play a day-to-day role in private practice; patients may see any psychiatrist they choose. A psychiatrist must perpetually demonstrate his or her effectiveness by expert evaluation and treatment of patients.

Those trying to build a practice with a substantial proportion of psychotherapy patients encounter special problems. For the initial several sessions, one must constantly be both therapist and teacher, helping the patient to see the value of psychotherapy in a compelling way. Furthermore, one must be alert to early negative transferences, a common cause for patients to discontinue treatment. During residency, observing and interpreting transferences, especially early ones that cause resistance in developing a working relationship, were a matter of intellectual interest and pleasing one's supervisor. In private practice, it is a matter of survival. Because referrals are precious, one must make the most of each patient who comes for help. Patients with severe trouble sustaining relationships will bring those troubles to the therapy relationship. Handling them adroitly may make the difference between patients who stay in therapy and improve their life and those who leave, diminished in hope and still dysfunctional.

Patterns of Referral

It is difficult to break established patterns of referral among doctors who have practiced together for decades. There is competition from other, nonphysician, mental health professionals who may have their own established networks of referrals. Many internists or family practitioners may prefer referring to a psychologist or social worker, rather than lose the patient to a psychiatrist who can take over complete management of the patient's illness. It is often unavoidable and appropriate for the psychiatrist to take over a patient's care. However, it is therefore understandable that the primary care doctor, who is competing to maintain his own patient load, may want to continue to see the patient and prescribe an anxiolytic while asking a social worker to do counseling.

A few measures can be taken to promote a healthier referral relationship with primary care physicians. First, select a few family practice or internal medicine physicians with whom you feel comfortable working and referring patients. Their suspicions of you will be relieved if you first become a source of referrals to them; you might even refer family or friends. They will then feel that they owe you the same courtesy and will send a patient to you. Don't be surprised if the first referrals are a "mess"; they will be the patients the referring physician wants to get rid of most. Patients may have been maintained on high doses of anxiolytics for years, or complicated depressions may have been treated with inadequate doses of antidepressants. Take care to not communicate to the patient that the referring physician has treated him or her inadequately and that he or she should have been sent to you much sooner. Unless the referring physician has been acting unethically, such communication serves no good purpose and will surely get back to the referring physician; that referral source will disappear. Instead, correct the treatment and, if necessary, gently educate the referring physician as to the change in treatment you have instituted and discuss both your continuing role and the referring physician's role in the patient's care.

Educating primary care physicians about psychiatric illness and appropriateness of referral is very helpful for practice development. This can easily spring from your position of unit chief in the hospital as you become involved with the continuing medical education activities of the hospital. You must remember that psychiatry is impenetrable to most primary care physicians. Ironically, it is most of what they see. Being seen as a resource, someone to bail them out of difficult situations and take on their difficult patients, while retaining a good working relationship with them, will facilitate developing and keeping your valuable sources of patient referral.

I may appear to be rather negative about how primary care physicians handle psychiatric patients. You may encounter physicians who appropriately refer the difficult patients with symptoms they cannot manage, and who competently treat patients with uncomplicated depression or transient anxiety they see daily. I am sure many such physicians are practicing, but in my experience they are the exceptions.

Social Skills

One of the most important assets for going into private practice is an engaging and gregarious personality. Having a desire to interact and socialize with other doctors on the hospital medical staff and generally fitting into their community are important in sustaining yourself in practice. Most psychiatrists are introverted. Other physicians are relieved when they meet a psychiatrist they can identify as an "ordinary Joe" (or Josephine) and who can talk to them without jargon. For example, one should say: "Mrs. Smith is very depressed and is thinking about hurting herself and needs to be in the hospital," not "Mrs. Smith is mourning the loss of her cat, which recapitulates the loss of her mother to whom she was ambivalent and whose negative introject is causing her self-hatred and thoughts of suicide." Other physicians already assume psychiatrists are weird; do not confirm it for them.

Psychiatrists in private practice must demonstrate their value to colleagues and patients. To colleagues, this is done through successful treatment of referred patients. It is very important that the referring physician does not hear complaints from patients referred to you about your work or demeanor. You must be reliable and available and make his or her patients grateful for the referral. You must communicate promptly with the referring physician, either verbally or in writing (preferably both), about your assessment and treatment plan. To patients, you demonstrate your value by expertly and ethically helping them to understand themselves in ways they could not do alone and by efficiently relieving their distressing symptoms.

Practice Partnerships

In the winter of 1983, I did not see a future of growth in my practice in the manner I was proceeding. I had to either take a job at a hospital or clinic, at a much reduced rate of compensation, or to form some type of partnership with someone.

My solution was to enter into a partnership. One of my colleagues had begun a practice the previous year in the suburbs and was very busy. He was interested in hospital practice, outpatient medication management, and supportive, structuring psychotherapy for sicker patients. I was interested primarily in outpatient short- and long-term psychodynamic psychotherapy. Our overlap was in covering the hospital practice on the weekends and covering for each other's vacations. Our skills and interests dovetailed perfectly, and each of us respected the other's work. For 10 years, my practice proceeded in this way; half of my time was spent downtown seeing private outpatients and psychoanalytic control cases, and the other half was spent in outpatient practice in our suburban office. Covering for my partner's hospital practice, I saw hospital patients on an addiction unit and a general psychiatric unit every other weekend. Interestingly, as time went on, many of my downtown patients originated from the suburban office. People who were initially seen where they lived (i.e., in the suburbs) were followed more conveniently where they worked (i.e., in the city). It was an interesting and productive partnership; our work paralleled each others, converging in weekend coverage and cross referring of patients according to which of our skills they needed.

For me, the city represented my psychoanalytic training; professional society involvement, including committee memberships and elected positions; and an outpatient practice of mostly longer-term, insight-oriented, psychodynamic psychotherapy patients. The suburbs represented more general psychiatric outpatient care and hospital work. The suburban practice involved seeing more family members. Downtown, you might see an insurance salesman; in the suburbs, you might see his wife, retired mother, or teenage children. You may initially treat the wife for anxiety attacks, but later see her and her husband for marriage counseling. The retired mother might have an endogenous depression or a substance abuse problem, and the teenager might have problems with adolescence. The level of competition for patients in the suburbs is less than in the city; the farther you are from an urban setting, the more psychiatric services are spread out.

In this setting, you structure your own work week. The standard schedule for a general practice is to see hospital patients in the morning and outpatients in the afternoon. This is sprinkled with a few hours of teaching, hospital committees, and phone calls. A part-time job may occupy a block of time in your schedule.

Patient care waxes and wanes in private practice. I used to joke with my partner: when the practice was hectic, it was miserable; when it was slow, it was miserable. The patient load never seems to be precisely what you want. It is very difficult to refuse work, for many reasons. However, psychiatric work can be quite stressful, and when one is overworked, it can be a real burden. Coping with these periods requires some character strength. Conversely, when the practice is quiet, and the hours begin to slip, you may begin to panic. You wonder when this declining trend will stop, if ever, and how to turn the practice around again. This also requires some character strength to weather.

After several years, this pattern of peaks and valleys becomes easier to tolerate as you realize that either phase eventually reverses. Some partnerships are less felicitous than mine was. A resident entering practice and considering becoming a junior partner or "employee" of an established practice has a continuum of opportunity. On one end of the scale, there is entry into a partnership in which the demand for psychiatric services in the community is high, and full integration into the practice is rapid if you perform well during the first year or two. Progress is rapid, because if you are not brought fully into the partnership quickly enough, you will soon realize that you will have more success by starting your own practice and competing with the practice that hired you and introduced you to the medical community. A partnership's success depends on the equity of the practice arrangements, the amiability of the personalities involved, and a mutual respect for the professional expertise and conduct among all the partners.

At the other end of the spectrum, more common in urban environments, is entry into a partnership of a large, hospital-based, assembly-line practice consisting of primarily chronic patients. Demand for psychiatric services in a large city is generally low because many mental health professionals are competing for patients. The patients treated in this type of hospital-based practice are usually receiving disability and may reside in nursing homes for chronically mentally ill patients. They are hospitalized when their symptoms become difficult to manage in the nursing home. This creates a revolving door pattern, with patients being shuttled between the nursing home and the hospital. The fees to the practice are based on how many hospital beds are kept filled at any given time. As many as a dozen such nursing homes may be used to funnel patients into the general psychiatric units of several hospitals, with each patient receiving only the most cursory care. In this practice, outpatient follow-up may be given short shrift.

This type of business is very lucrative, and several psychiatrists may be necessary to service all the beds involved. You may be hired for that function. It is difficult to get out of this type of practice. There is no opportunity to develop an alternative practice, because you are so busy with the patients from the nursing homes. Of course, chronically mentally ill patients in the inner city are an underserved population that require more psychiatric services. I am not suggesting avoiding practicing in that setting. Providing good quality psychiatric care to that population is vital. However, it is not a common career path in the urban setting. Becoming employed by such a practice can be a discouraging and costly lesson that can set your career back a couple of years.

Partnership contracts. Although I did not have a partnership contract, I think my situation was unusual. In our partnership, neither of us was dispensable. It was a very equal situation and worked to our mutual benefit. However, I would not neglect having a contract again. A contract is essential, especially when one is starting out in practice, when the positions are unequal. Ask psychiatrists in your area what type of contract they have, what pitfalls they encountered, and who draws up contracts. Find an attorney who has done such work before, possibly through a colleague who had a successful experience with the attorney.

You should look for many elements in a partnership contract. This list is by no means exhaustive; it only represents certain highlights.

- Ensure that the obvious points of salary, hours, vacation, benefits, and call schedule are satisfactory to you and competitive for that locale.
- If possible, make certain that eligibility for full, equal partnership is part of the contract, with a definite time frame, usually 2 or 3 years.
- Be aware of the presence of a clause that may forbid you from practicing in the immediate area if you leave the partnership.
- Ask about certain contingencies, such as how much vacation your employing psychiatrist will take, leaving you to manage the entire practice. Also, determine who will take off which holidays.
- Ask about any malpractice or ethics proceedings against your prospective employer. If possible, when visiting the office and hospital, review a handful of charts to see the level of documentation; sloppy charts invite malpractice judgments, and you will be sharing malpractice liability with the other psychiatrist(s) in the practice whose patients you cover. Remember, if your signature appears on the chart, you are likely to be named in any suit, whether or not you were actually involved.
- Make sure you are comfortable with the clinical skills of your prospective partner(s).

Changing Career Paths

After 10 years in partnership, I became restless. I was tired of commuting to the suburbs, I was becoming bored, and I felt that I was not growing professionally. Although my practice was quite successful, I had anxiety about the prospect of looking out of my office window for the rest of my life with nothing more to look forward to. I wanted to find a way to bring my practice downtown full time and to enhance my professional life. It would have been much easier to make the opposite transition and move out to the suburbs full time, because that is where most of the business was. However, my wife worked downtown and my children went to private school downtown, so I wanted to move the practice there.

This time, as I approached "re-entering" full-time practice downtown, I felt more knowledgeable and better prepared. I looked at the several private hospitals downtown to decide which were the best candidates for my practice. I was looking for a good quality institution, perhaps a teaching hospital, where the psychiatrists were not "crawling over each other" competing for referrals. Only a couple of hospitals fit that description. At one, the director of inpatient services was an instructor from my residency program. I called him to inquire about the practice opportunities. It was coincidental that I called. They had opened a small inpatient unit, emphasizing a psychodynamic approach to higher functioning patients, and were looking for a quarter-time unit director. In retrospect, this is something I might have done 10 years earlier, but conditions were really quite different. Now, I had 10 years of experience treating all types of psychiatric patients, I had been through a period of psychoanalytic training, and I had some administrative experience from hospital committees and the local district branch of the American Psychiatric Association.

I had hoped this position would provide an immediate entry into the medical staff, a small supplement to my income to help make up for the loss caused by leaving the suburban office, and a source of referrals for my office practice. It accomplished all three to various degrees, and, as a bonus, I discovered that I enjoyed the administrative side of the work. Although I had done some administrative work in other settings, I had not had full administrative responsibility for anything. This made the work a challenge and a good antidote for the restlessness I was beginning to feel after 10 years of only seeing patients.

After a year and a half as director of the inpatient unit, I was asked to administer the hospital's multidisciplinary outpatient psychiatric clinic. This was a half-time position and involved contact with and supervision of professionals in other mental health disciplines.

I settled into a routine of working at the psychiatric clinic in the morning, assigning patients who had called that day to therapists, monitoring the quality of the ongoing treatment plans for the clinic's therapists, supervising students and residents, seeing an occasional private consultation or inpatient, and performing various teaching functions for the department. In the afternoon, I would go to my private office several blocks away and see my private outpatients.

I had expectations for advancement in the administrative aspect of my work, either within the department in which I was working or at another institution. One advantage of working in an urban center is the sheer number of opportunities available. I discovered that it was very important to me to have the prospect of something more—a new professional challenge to obsess about and look forward to.

Managed Care

During the 1980s, sweeping changes affected the way clinical practice was conducted in all of areas of medicine. From the practitioners' perspective, the most striking and disturbing change has been the decline in autonomy of individual physicians. Managed care has brought with it the third-party micromanagement of individual cases. Some large psychiatric managed care companies see themselves as managing the actual care delivered and not the benefits structure. Autonomy in judgment, using consultation when necessary, has been the hallmark of private medical practice and a major inducement for talented, independent, and bright young men and women to enter the field. Managed care has "hatcheted" into that autonomy. Sound medical judgment used to be the driving force behind the standard of psychiatric care; now it is fiscal restraint and second guessing managed care employees whose profit is based on denying benefits and who never have to face the patient. The individual practicing physician has little control over these events.

In 1982, when I entered general psychiatric practice, there was essentially no third-party management of private medical care. The Peer Review Improvement Act of 1982 [Part B, Title XI, Social Security Act Section 1154 (a)(7)(c)] required Medicare providers to release patient medical record information to private reviewers before payment. A multitude of third-party medical review organizations materialized to oversee the quality and necessity of medical care delivered.

I thought that the whole point of my medical school and residency training was to train me to make autonomous clinical decisions and to know when to seek consultation. Like many of my peers, I was outraged when the first nurse practitioner called me on the telephone so that I could present my patient's case to her and hope for authorization of 3 days of hospital care; I had to justify my clinical decisions again to be granted an additional 3 days. It seemed like the practice of medicine had turned upside down. For practical purposes, to limit payment for care is to limit care itself. Those deciding the limits of care were, it seemed to me, untrained, and their blatant motive was to profit from the limitation of care. Over the past 10 years, I have become more sophisticated about how managed care companies work, and the third-party management of medical care is becoming more sophisticated and standardized.

My initial perception was that managed care reviewers were interested in reducing costs without regard to quality of care. However, in recent years they have seemed increasingly to identify themselves as members of the treatment team, with the role of ensuring cost-effective and well-considered care in the least restrictive environment. For example, one major managed care company recently sought consultation from our state medical society to ensure that its guidelines for medical necessity were congruent with local accepted standards of practice.

In dealing with reviewers, I have found several principles to be very helpful. First, accept that they are an unavoidable part of the health care system, and keep your rage or resentment out of the conversation. Second, describe in everyday, common-sense terms the functional impairment that makes hospitalization (for example) necessary for the patient, how the treatment plan addresses this impairment, and what changes must occur before the patient can be discharged responsibly. Descriptions limited to diagnosis and symptoms do not adequately address the concerns of utilization review. Details of how to communicate and document the need for treatment can be found in *Managing Managed Care: A Mental Health Practitioner's Survival Guide* (Goodman et al. 1992), a book that I have found very helpful in dealing with managed care reviewers.

If the first-level reviewer denies payment, the appeal process (in which you talk to a physician) is likely to be more successful. Relatively few psychiatrists take the time to appeal, and I have found that managed care companies take such an effort seriously. The fact that there have now been successful suits against such companies when patients have committed suicide after premature discharge has made them more reluctant to deny payment for care that a psychiatrist insists is absolutely necessary. On some occasions, I have even received approval for long-term, intensive psychotherapy when I could prove that it was a viable alternative to hospitalization and documented ongoing functional improvement.

One aspect of managed care for which there is no remedy is the amount of administrative time required to meet the review criteria for the managed care company. In a larger group practice, a designated employee may handle the early stages of review. If you are alone, or with one or two other partners, managed care reviews steal considerable time away from patient care. My initial approach of rage at the reviewer was not particularly useful; learning the managed care drill and getting through it as quickly as possible is the best one can do.

When entering into a managed care contract, read the fine print and try to imagine how the terms of the contract will affect everyday practice and difficulties that may arise. Your lawyer can help you better understand the legal implications of the contract's language. Phrases such as "the physician shall retain full clinical responsibility for the management of the patient" may sound like a statement of faith in the doctor's abilities, but may actually be included to assign *liability* to the doctor, rather than responsibility.

Another concern is the fee structure. How is it established and when is it renegotiated? How are referrals to specialists made? Are they discouraged? Do the gatekeepers get paid more if they refer less? What are the criteria for medical necessity for hospitalization or outpatient treatment? What are their customary limitations on length of care? What happens when the benefits stop, but the patient requires further care? These questions are the tip of the iceberg to understanding a managed care contract, so read carefully and seek legal advice if you are uncertain about exactly what you are being asked to sign.

To what extent is it possible to avoid managed care in an urban practice? In my current part-time practice, I see relatively few managed care patients. This stems from having gradually built up a caseload of people who can pay for psychotherapy largely out of their own pockets. Although it is no longer realistic to expect to fill up a full-time practice with such patients, a psychiatrist in my area who has built a good referral network for 10 to 15 years might be able to fill 25% to 50% of his or her hours with self-pay patients. Of course, this would not be true for psychiatrists who specialize in inpatient treatment.

The Future of Urban Practice

It is difficult to discuss at this time the future of urban psychiatric practice when we appear to be on the brink of precipitous changes in medical practice, mandated by the government. The two major systems of medical care delivery being debated are managed competition versus a single-payer system. Managed competition is a system in which large corporations with their thousands of employees would accept competitive bids for the provision of health care services offered by large groups of competing health care providers. This system would probably not allow for, or at least would discourage, the existence of successful private office practice in the urban setting. All patients with third-party reimbursement would be directed to the large group providers. In urban settings, these group providers would be large indeed, composed of networks of hospitals and their medical staffs. These networks are already forming in the large urban areas. These groups would manage themselves, providing services at a low enough cost to be able to bid competitively with the other networks of providers. The solo practitioner gets squeezed out of this process.

The other option is a single-payer system, similar to the one in Canada. In this system, taxes would form the "insurance premium" and the government would pay the bills. Under this system, solo practice could survive, although standards of medical care and reimbursement schedules would be fixed by the government.

One possible contingency in the single-payer system that would allow psychoanalysis and long-term psychotherapy to survive would be to authorize private independent contracting with physicians, parallel to, but separate from, the government single-payer system, as in Great Britain.

Current financial pressures are causing most psychiatrists to function in an even more limited way. In an HMO, the psychiatrist's role in patient care is limited to medication evaluation and management. Psychotherapy is done by social workers or other lower paid therapists. This trend could make psychiatry less attractive to medical students at a time when enrollment in psychiatric residency training is at a low, leading to an exodus away from urban psychiatric practice to other settings. However, the attraction of urban practice has withstood intense competition, managed care, and decreasing patient base. Evolving changes in urban practice patterns as a result of upcoming government health care reform are yet to be seen. The urban setting offers such a wide variety of practice opportunities that it is likely to remain the most popular setting for psychiatric practice throughout the 1990s.

References

Dorwart RA, Chartock LR, Dial T, et al: A national study of psychiatrists' professional activities. Am J Psychiatry 149:1499–1505, 1992

Goodman M, Brown J, Dietz P (eds): Managing Managed Care: A Mental Health Practitioners Survival Guide. Washington, DC, American Psychiatric Press, 1992

Chapter 3

Small-City Psychiatric Practice

Dominic Mazza, M.D.

*I*n this chapter, I focus on the characteristics of private psychiatric practice in a small city—Scranton, Pennsylvania. As of the 1990 census, the population of this city was 81,805. Scranton is in Lackawanna County, the northeastern part of Pennsylvania. The total population of Lackawanna County (Scranton and its surrounding communities) is approximately 220,000. This city is typical of many in the northeastern United States that have seen considerable declines in population over the past few decades. Scranton's heyday was in the early to middle decades of this century when coal mining and steel production were vibrant economic forces. As these industries grew less viable, a corresponding diminution in the population ensued.

A strong ethnic presence exists in this community, primarily Italian, Polish, Irish, and Jewish second- and third-generation western European emigrants who settled here during the late nineteenth and early twentieth century. Church and family remain a vital influence for much of the community. This gives Scranton more of a small-town flavor than its population would suggest. These factors are of considerable importance to the practice of psychiatry in this community. The psychiatrist's presence in this community is much more visible, and, more importantly, one's personal as well as therapeutic successes and failures are readily apparent to the community at large. Indeed, community norms and expectations may define therapeutic success quite differently from treating physicians or their patients. For example, a patient's decision to divorce may be viewed quite differently by the community than by the patient and/or the therapist.

Background

I am a board-certified psychiatrist, and I am certified in adult, adolescent, and child psychoanalysis by the American Psychoanalytic Association. Before settling in Scranton, I was an air force psychiatrist and a faculty member of the Uniform Services University of the Health Sciences, Bethesda, Maryland. I chose Scranton to establish a practice for several reasons, including proximity to family, fewer of the pressures that plague large urban centers, and an atmosphere that my wife and I believed would be beneficial to our children.

Several psychiatrists have practiced in this city; 10 psychiatrists are currently in private practice in Scranton itself, but at least 5 of these spend the bulk of their time in salaried institutional work and see few private patients. To my knowledge, a trained psychoanalyst has never practiced in this area. I continue to be the only analyst within a 100-mile radius from this community, a fact that was of considerable importance to me as I contemplated settling here.

My professional interests are varied, but my primary focus is psychoanalysis. In addition, I have always been interested in psychosomatic medicine. This location has allowed me to pursue both of these interests as well as other areas of practice that I only serendipitously developed as a result of this move.

In anticipation of my move to this area, I faced many of the concerns that confront any physician about to establish a practice in a new community. These concerns included questions about the financial viability of a new practice in a new location, the challenge of introducing and integrating oneself into an established medical and psychiatric community, and the unique variables that affect hospital privileges and specific third-party payer policies idiosyncratic to each state or city. My solution to these potential problems was to first secure a part-time salaried position that would give me time to familiarize myself with the vagaries of private practice in Scranton.

Initiating a Practice Through Consultation Psychiatry

Scranton itself is served by three acute care hospitals; there is only one 40-bed inpatient psychiatric unit. As I investigated psychiatric practice in Scranton before my move, it became clear to me that a consultation-liaison service was desperately needed, as none existed. I discussed this with several psychiatrists who were in practice in Scranton, and, although a few did psychiatric consultations for medical or surgical patients on a limited basis, they all underscored the need for more formal consultation-liaison services. As a result of these discussions, I met with the chief of psychiatry at the community hospital that had the inpatient psychiatric unit. We agreed that I would establish a consultation-liaison section of this department to serve the three hospitals in the community. This satisfied my interest in psychosomatic medicine, helped to integrate me into the medical community, and, of course, assuaged any immediate financial concerns.

Within several weeks of my move to Scranton, the consultation-liaison service developed into an integral part of the department of psychiatry and generated more requests for psychiatric consultation than one part-time psychiatrist could ever conceivably satisfy. As one might expect, my presence on medical/surgical and pediatric wards of the three city hospitals served as an excellent avenue into the medical community, which then led to an ever-expanding source of referrals from nonpsychiatric physicians for outpatient psychiatric evaluation and treatment.

The significant lesson from this experience is the vital importance of integrating oneself within the established medical community, especially with our nonpsychiatric colleagues. Joining the local medical society is not enough; one needs to be an intimate partner in the care of patients outside of a strictly psychiatric setting. Unfortunately, many psychiatrists and certainly the majority of psychoanalyst physicians seem to have forgotten or ignored this lesson during the past few decades.

Characteristics of a
Small-City Practice Psychiatrist

Currently, my professional hours are allocated as follows: 15 to 20 hours per week—psychiatric consultation to medical/surgical/pediatric units; 30 to 35 hours per week—psychoanalysis/psychotherapy; 5 to 10 hours per week—supervision/administration. I do not provide direct care for inpatients in the psychiatric unit in our city, but I do provide occasional consultation. I do not participate in any organizations such as health maintenance organizations (HMOs) or preferred provider organizations (PPOs), although they are increasingly common in Scranton as throughout the United States. (I have provided treatment on a "case by case" basis to patients who have been in these programs and will describe some details later in this chapter.) Coverage limits for outpatient treatment vary widely from policy to policy; almost all of my patients assume responsibility for a significant portion (usually 50%) of the fee for my services. Of course, as has long been the tradition in psychiatry, I see a number of patients at adjusted fees commensurate with their financial resources. My experience in this location has been that I and other psychiatrists, who provide sound psychodynamically oriented therapy and medication management, have had much less trouble maintaining a full practice than those who only prescribe medication. My impression is that psychotherapeutic expertise can help psychiatrists to maintain a full practice without depending on referrals from managed care organizations.

Some aspects of a small-city practice are specific to my identity as a psychoanalyst/psychiatrist. These primarily concern educating non-psychiatrist physicians and the community at large about psychoanalysis: clarifying its role, value, and limitations, and correcting common misconceptions (i.e., "It is only for the idle rich," "You only talk about sex and your mother," "It lasts a lifetime," a la Woody Allen!).

Yet, I believe that for the most part, my experience generalizes easily to any psychiatrist interested in establishing a successful practice in a small city. However, I stress that this applicability refers to the establishment of a primarily outpatient practice. Given the current political-medical-economic climate in which inpatient psychiatric care is subject to considerable scrutiny, at times driven by strictly financial concerns, the ability to care for patients outside of an inpatient psychiatric hospital setting is increasingly becoming the sine qua non of a successful private psychiatric practice.

Many patients can be successfully treated for their Axis I disorders in outpatient programs that utilize pharmacotherapy and more supportive psychotherapies. In my clinical experience, however, a considerable subgroup of patients with Axis I disorders exists whose symptomatology and treatments are complicated by significant character pathology (i.e., Axis II disorders). This group of patients has a less than satisfactory response to pharmacotherapy and/or supportive psychotherapies. Also, brief inpatient stays on acute care psychiatric units have not proven to be effective interventions in many of these patients. In my experience, these patients' symptoms are more effectively managed in more intensive psychotherapeutic treatment based on sound psychodynamic principles. Thus, once again, my identity as a psychotherapist/psychoanalyst has played a major role in establishing a successful practice.

Advantages of a Small-City Practice

Now, I would like to discuss some advantages of a small-city practice. Of course, practicing in a community of this size allows one to become more familiar with the resources available to support and enhance psychiatric treatment than would be possible in a larger city. Clearly, it is immeasurably easier to become familiar with community mental health centers, vocational rehabilitation programs, child protective services, and other community support services in a city with 80,000 people than in one with several million. This is a considerable benefit in one's continual need to mobilize community resources to facilitate all aspects of psychiatric treatment and rehabilitation.

Compared with those practicing in large metropolitan areas, the small-city psychiatrist is more likely to meet and become acquainted with those people who hold positions of power and influence in all sections of the community (e.g., judicial, educational, financial, religious, and political). The psychiatrist practicing in this setting can potentially bring mental health concerns to the attention of those individuals exerting the most influence in the community. For instance, I was introduced socially to the county district attorney; we then met at other community events. Ultimately, areas of mutual professional interest became topics of cocktail party conversation or chance sidewalk visits. Within a short time he invited me to have lunch to discuss his office's handling of child sexual abuse investigations and to request consultation and in-service training for his staff.

On another occasion, I had the fortuitous experience of hearing a pastor of a large parish address his congregation on the evils of our "overtherapized society" and the need "to return to Jesus for help." Shortly thereafter, I had an opportunity to invite him to breakfast; of course, I raised my concerns about the potential pernicious effects of his well-intentioned remarks about therapy. We had a fruitful and mutually beneficial discussion about "faith and Freud"; he has become a strong supporter of mental health services and an important avenue to direct many members of the community to receive the psychiatric treatment they need and deserve.

In a smaller city, the practicing psychiatrist is much more likely to become acquainted with members of the business community, ranging from independent businesspeople or small-business owners to leaders of local industry. A distinct advantage inherent in a community this size is the opportunity to be a positive force influencing both the environment of the workplace and the employer's support for equitable coverage for psychiatric illness. These are only a few of the myriad examples of the benefits of small-city professional intimacies. In a large metropolitan area, a given psychiatrist will also have some similar professional acquaintances, but not the potential impact on his community afforded to the psychiatrist in a smaller urban area.

In a smaller city, only a few judges are involved in areas of concern to psychiatrists. For instance, in Scranton, one judge adjudicates at family court. There are two city public high schools and a few private ones. Consequently, in this environment, a practicing psychiatrist has the potential to know high school principals and counselors, as well as school board members. Within 1 year of beginning my practice, I was invited to serve as a board member for the Northeastern Pennsylvania Tri-County Mental Health/Mental Retardation Board of Directors, and I have since served as the chairman of the Mental Health Subcommittee.

From this vantage point, one has the opportunity to become acquainted with the manner in which federal, state, and local mental health dollars are allocated and to have some influence on this process. In a large city, one would not be as privy to so comprehensive a view and would not usually be able to influence the utilization of mental health resources throughout one's community.

Another distinct advantage in a small city, at this time, is considerably less interference from managed care personnel. Because of the small population and because the pool of professionals is also smaller, managed care organizations are by necessity staffed by a limited number of "managers"; thus, psychiatrists can develop a professional/working alliance with some of those administrators. This allows for greater negotiating flexibility than would ever exist in large cities. In my experience, if one can convincingly demonstrate the financial savings that intensive outpatient treatment offers to selected patients, managed care organizations are much more willing to support such treatment on a case-by-case basis. For example, I have secured support for psychoanalytic treatment of patients whose coverage would only support inpatient care and who were at risk of requiring hospitalization if outpatient treatment of sufficient intensity was not supported by the case manager.

A number of clinicians had treated one patient for an eating disorder over the course of several months, which included inpatient psychiatric treatment. I was consulted during a period of worsening symptoms when inpatient hospitalization was again imminent. The case manager agreed to support an intensive outpatient program "to avoid further hospitalizations." Because the outcome was successful, the organization managing this patient's care has been more willing to support intensive outpatient treatment for other patients. I have had similar experiences with other managed care organizations.

I am not implying that there is now broad-based support for psychoanalysis or intensive psychotherapies, but rather that if one can demonstrate to third-party payers that these treatments are financially advantageous in particular cases, then one may be able to garner support for these treatments. Similarly, I am not suggesting that psychiatrists practicing in small cities have no disputes with managed care administrators, but that the potential exists for establishing ongoing personal working relationships, which can benefit both our patients and the organizations that help support their treatment.

I believe that these examples demonstrate some of the interesting aspects and distinct advantages of a small-city practice. Alas! There is no free lunch. Now, I present some of the challenges and potential difficulties of small-city psychiatric practices.

Disadvantages of a Small-City Practice

One clear disadvantage of a small-city practice is a limited supply of trained and experienced clinicians to whom one might refer patients. As I mentioned earlier in this chapter, I am the only trained psychoanalyst within a few hours' drive. Consequently, anyone interested in an analysis (and there are more than a few) or anyone whose neurotic or characterological difficulties would be amenable only to a full psychoanalytic process (and there are many more) have only two options: me, or travel more than 100 miles in each direction several times per week. Needless to say, for the vast majority of patients the latter option is not feasible. Under these circumstances, one must, by necessity, reassess the ideal of anonymity balanced with the needs of the patient.

Many psychiatrists, and certainly the vast majority of psychoanalysts, have been taught that the anonymity of the clinician is an important, useful, and, quite possibly, essential ingredient in the therapeutic process. I am well aware of a theoretical continuum that ranges from those clinicians who view self-disclosure by the therapist as not interfering in their treatment of patients to those who hold the therapist's anonymity as sacrosanct and necessary for effective treatment. In a small-city practice, the practicing psychiatrist, perforce, is much more likely to be someone many of his patients have knowledge about to various degrees. This is not secondary to the clinician's theoretical position on anonymity, but related to the realities of small-city life. Strikingly little has been written in the psychoanalytic and psychiatric literature on this inescapable aspect of practice in a small city.

A few psychoanalytic articles have addressed extra-analytical contacts between analyst and patient, and these are considered "special events." These articles do not discuss the particular setting (e.g., a small city), which, by definition, creates a perturbation in the anonymity or transference balance (Greenacre 1959; Tarnower 1966; Weiss 1975). Freud (1905/1981a, 1909/1981b) described some effects of his patients' "outside" knowledge about him, but these descriptions were early case material before he had fully appreciated and articulated the centrality of transference elaboration and exploration. A recent issue of the journal *Psychotherapy in Private Practice* has focused on the practice of psychotherapy in rural communities; although these articles address some similar concerns about anonymity and "dual relationships," rural practice experience does not easily transfer to small-city practice (Sobel 1992; Sterling 1992).

This dilemma, although of significant importance to a psychoanalyst, is of no small concern to the general psychiatrist in a small city either. We do not know, for instance, what impact significant knowledge about one's psychopharmacologist's personal life (foibles and successes) might have on medication treatment, or how details of a psychiatrist's divorce might affect the outcome of marital therapy. With a more limited referral network than is available in a large metropolis, the small-city psychiatrist is much more likely to face these therapeutic questions and dilemmas, and, at times, this potential complication does not surface until treatment is well underway.

In a small city, not only the anonymity of the psychiatrist is compromised. Patients and potential patients are likely to know considerably more about the psychiatrist's colleagues, staff, and family members than most of us might have experienced during professional training, which usually takes place in larger cities. Indeed, the psychiatrist may also know significant details about a patient, the patient's family, and his or her colleagues. In this context, transference expression is potentially complicated, and countertransference pressures are certainly colored by "outside" knowledge about one's patients and their significant others.

Issues of confidentiality become more problematic in a small city. In my practice, I do not use an answering service, but rather a telephone answering machine, because in a small city, there is a much greater likelihood that patients would be recognized by the answering service personnel. Patients can also be easily recognized and identified by pedestrians or other patients while entering or leaving one's office. Some psychiatrists arrange their own appointments and do their own billing (I am one); others feel more comfortable with their staff handling these aspects of psychiatric practice.

I have established some professional guidelines that might not be necessary in larger cities, and I have had to balance my responsibilities to the community with those to my family. I will not see friends of my children or members of their class at school or friends of my wife or their family members. In a large city, this would not be such a dilemma, because there are always other professionals to whom one can refer these patients. In a smaller city with more limited referral sources, another clinician, with the specific expertise and training required to treat a particular patient, may not be available.

This leads to another dilemma: where does one turn for consultation, supervision, or therapy, given the potential professional isolation and peculiar countertransference pressures of a small-city practice? In Philadelphia, New York City, San Francisco, or similar locations, the possibilities are legion; in a small city, they may be scarce or nonexistent. My involvement in the local, state, and national psychiatric societies and my work within a psychoanalytic institute and with psychoanalytic colleagues have been restorative and essential.

In addition, my practice in Scranton has evolved to include a considerable amount of supervision of local psychotherapists, both private practitioners and institutional caregivers (i.e., therapists employed at community clinics or residential treatment facilities). I had not thought much about this aspect of practice prior to settling here, but I have found it to be both challenging and rewarding. When I first began my practice here, it took some time for me to clarify which roles I would be willing to assume in my collaborative work with other mental health professionals. I will provide consultation with clinicians wishing to discuss a particular therapeutic dilemma or see their patients for consultation should the treating therapist believe it to be of potential value. I refuse to see another mental health professional's patient until this is discussed and explored with the treating clinician. To do otherwise, I believe, is professionally unethical and a disservice to both the patient and clinician. I expect other professionals to be as judicious, and I have not found this to be a problem.

I have not been willing to provide psychopharmacological treatment of patients in treatment with nonpsychiatric mental health care providers. Some of these providers have found this stance problematic; others have understood and been supportive. I have decided on this posture for many reasons: 1) a number of general psychiatrists in the area have psychopharmacological expertise that certainly equals or surpasses mine; 2) I believe my working hours are better spent providing primary clinical care of patients or providing supervision; and 3) I have serious concerns about the course many of our psychiatric colleagues have charted, namely primarily providing psychopharmacological management and abdicating psychotherapeutic treatment of adults and children to nonpsychiatrists.

Some colleagues express concern that they must maintain their practices by providing "psychopharmacological backup" to nonpsychiatric mental health care providers as a result of the competitive pressure. I have not found this to be the case. Although I consider psychopharmacological consultation to be a valuable service provided by psychiatrists to the communities they serve, I would argue that psychiatrists with solid clinical skills that include psychotherapeutic expertise will not find themselves relegated to the role of "medication provider" by economic necessity.

Conclusion

I have found the small-city practice to be an interesting, challenging, and rewarding opportunity. Most counties in the United States are underserved by psychiatrists; consequently, there is a dire clinical imperative for more psychiatrists to consider practicing outside large urban communities and academic settings. In addition to the considerable benefits of a small-city lifestyle, there are abundant professional rewards and challenges. I have not been disappointed.

References

Freud S: Fragment of an analysis of a case of hysteria (1905), in The Standard Edition of the Complete Psychological Works of Sigmund Freud, Vol 7. Translated and edited by Strachey J. London, Hogarth Press, 1981a, pp 7–122

Freud S: Notes upon a case of obsessional neurosis (1909), in The Standard Edition of the Complete Psychological Works of Sigmund Freud, Vol 10. Translated and edited by Strachey J. London, Hogarth Press, 1981b, pp 155–318

Greenacre P: Certain technical problems in the transference relationship. J Am Psychoanal Assoc 7:484–502, 1959

Sobel S: Small town practice of psychotherapy: ethical and personal dilemmas. Psychotherapy in Private Practice 10:61–69, 1992

Sterling DL: Practicing rural psychotherapy: complexity of role and boundary. Psychotherapy in Private Practice 10:105–127, 1992

Tarnower W: Extra-analytic contacts between the psychoanalyst and the patient. Psychoanal Q 35:399–413, 1966

Weiss S: The effect on the transference of "special events" occurring during psychoanalysis. Int J Psychoanal 56:69–75, 1975

Chapter 4

Rural Psychiatric Practice

David van Dyke, M.D.

*L*iving in a rural area and developing a private psychiatric practice has been part conscious decision and part fortuitous circumstance for me. In this chapter, I will try to describe the development of my practice in the public and private sectors, personal values that have influenced my decision, some impacts of rural life on myself and my family, and issues that I believe are common for anyone considering a rural practice.

Deciding to Practice in a Rural Area

I first made the decision to practice in a rural area while choosing a psychiatric residency. During medical school, I became aware that I did not want to live in a big city even for the few years of a residency. I also realized that I did not want to do research. This was a significant change in directions for me. I had entered medical school with an undergraduate biochemistry background, with plans for a Ph.D. in biochemistry and a research career. During medical school, I realized that I liked the intellectual challenge of research but really enjoyed working with people. I surprised myself by thoroughly enjoying my psychiatry rotation. It seemed to combine my enjoyment of being with people with an application of biochemistry through the growing understanding of psychobiology and psychopharmacology.

I selected Winnebago Mental Health Institute in Wisconsin for my residency, in a program in which much of the second year would be in rural community mental health centers, and the consultation rotations could be in smaller rural hospitals. During residency, I liked the variety of patient problems and seeing patients presenting with no previous workup, which is typical in rural practice. There was also great opportunity to see medical problems that present psychiatrically. Patients were not usually seen by several medical specialists before seeing a psychiatrist as seemed to be the case in a medical-school setting. I continue to enjoy that aspect of a rural psychiatry practice and find that to be common in other rural practices.

During the rotations in the rural counties, I was informed of the urgent need for psychiatric consultation in those areas. Administrators of the community mental health centers where I worked asked me to moonlight, and I agreed to moonlight for 2 years in the rural counties. They began immediately recruiting for time after residency. Since that time and during all my years in rural psychiatric practice, I have found that there is always much more demand for psychiatric time than there are psychiatrists to fill it. Competition for patients is not an issue in rural areas.

As I neared completion of residency, my wife's and children's needs became more important. My wife and I met during my first year in medical school, were married just before the third year, and by the end of my training, had two children. We also moved four times during medical school and residency. At that point, my wife and I felt the need to find a community and settle down, at least for a large block of our children's early school years, if that could be at all compatible with my practice interests.

Selecting a Location and Position

I began looking at options with community mental health clinics in western Wisconsin. We loved that area from visits there during residency. It is beautiful country and unique geologically. It is the only area in the Midwest that is unglaciated through all the past four ice ages! There are high ridges with well-kept dairy farms and contoured fields intermixed with steep hillsides forested with hardwoods. The area is about one-half farmland and one-half woodland and has a tremendous variety and abundance of wildlife. The communities are small and family oriented, and the farms are mostly single-family units. The terrain is just too broken for huge agribusiness operations. There are strong community feelings and strong support for the schools. The strong sense of local concern and control is reflected in the mental health system in Wisconsin. Each county has a community health clinic to ensure reasonable access. Clinics provide most of the services of the federal Community Mental Health Act, but often contract for hospital services.

A number of other rural positions were available in Wisconsin and adjacent midwestern states, and I was impressed that most were willing to be flexible and accommodate the goals of any psychiatrist interested in rural practice. I ultimately contracted to provide 20 hours per week of psychiatric services to the clinic in Vernon County. We bought a small farm outside Viroqua (the county seat), a town of about 3,500 people. The situation seemed to meet many of our needs. We found a community that would provide economic stability, if not affluence, and that was oriented toward education and development of responsibility in young people. Although definitely rural, the county is reasonably close to large population centers. Viroqua is 45 minutes from LaCrosse, a community that has two hospitals with psychiatric units and a university. It is 2 hours from Madison, with a major university, psychiatric residency program, and other advantages of a large university community.

Characteristics of the Rural Clinic

The mental health clinic in Vernon County had many characteristics that seemed to match my professional goals. I wanted a significant degree of autonomy in practice and an influence on clinic procedures, because I have clear standards for my practice and for those with whom I work and am responsible for. I also am unwilling to work in a system that focuses on rules or bureaucracy, especially if they are arbitrary and if they inhibit providing services to patients.

The clinic in Vernon County was just beginning, so the opportunity to develop the system was attractive. The three other staff members—a social worker with a master's degree, a psychiatric nurse, and a half-time psychologist—were all experienced, energetic, and able to function independently to a large degree. I believe the choice of these individuals reflected community values. The clinic was established as a nonprofit organization contracted with the county, rather than as a county-run clinic. This suggested an openness to independence and possibly innovation and gave a clear message of freedom from the bulk of county policies, procedures, and especially employment conditions, which are typically not acceptable to professionals.

Having a half-time position gave me the option to develop a private practice. No protective attitude existed to prevent me from doing so, even if I established a practice within the community. These conditions seemed to meet my need to establish a quality practice and be reasonably unencumbered by a bureaucracy.

Acceptance in a Rural Community

There are many levels of becoming accepted in a new community, and I think there are some additional ones for acceptance as a professional. There is an initial automatic and rather superficial acceptance granted because of your degree. However, in rural areas this is quite temporary, because rural people commonly distrust outsiders and "titles" or "ranks." Anyone hoping to be part of the community must demonstrate an ability to help both systems and individuals. In general, there is fairly tentative respect even from the medical community. I think my experience is fairly typical. I was the first medical specialist to move to the area. Initially, the family doctors appeared to be somewhat intimidated by the specialty status, but, at the same time, I felt the strong sentiment that I was not a "real" doctor. Despite that, initial consults were in the area of somatic problems and diagnostic help with neurology (i.e., "Is this someone who needs to see a neurologist?"). Later referrals were for more common psychiatric problems, such as severe depression and panic disorder. In rural practice, I found that it is important to take a very educational and supportive approach in all contacts with the physician community. In many rural areas, treatment of mental health problems is at best primitive, but noting the positive fosters open communication. Behavioral principles of "progressive approximation" and reinforcement of appropriate behavior work with caregivers as well as patients. It was also clear in my situation, as in any rural area I am aware of, that there will never be enough psychiatric time to care for all psychiatric issues. The family physician will care for many patients with mental health problems. The psychiatrist must remember that he or she is a consultant to family physicians and all other providers in a community.

Acceptance by the medical community is improved by participation in medical staff meetings and attendance at a reasonable amount of social events. After 5 years, I was elected chief of staff. I accepted the position, not because I enjoy that type of work, but because it represented the physicians' acceptance of me and my specialty.

The understanding of psychiatry as a medical specialty is minimal or nonexistent in many rural areas. This had an adverse economic consequence for me after a few months, when I went to the local bank to get a loan for a small private practice. I was turned down. I had no equity, only educational debt, and the specialty training had no value to the bank! Shortly thereafter, others explained my training in a medical specialty to the banker, and I opened my own office. During the next several years, I contracted most of my time in Vernon County, but consulted in two adjacent counties and continued the private practice. That initial time in part-time private practice was valuable to maintain psychotherapy skills and to develop experience with third-party payers and business issues.

Development of the Clinic

During the first year at the clinic in Vernon County, all staff members worked to establish the mental health clinic. We did a lot of public speaking about the availability of services in the county, the nature of mental health problems, and especially about treatment of major mental illness. We discovered a strong positive value that even though "we don't understand those problems," "we take care of our own." There was a strong and fairly extensive system of indigenous support for many mentally ill patients. It lacked many aspects of an appropriate treatment program and often had inappropriate or nonexistent medication management, but it was a resource to be developed.

The value of treating local patients by local doctors was strongly shared by those of us in the clinic, so we requested consultation concerning assertive community treatment as a new approach for treating chronically mentally ill patients, which was being developed at Mendota Mental Health Institute in Madison. We became the first county to modify these concepts for a rural area, and I implemented similar programs in the adjacent counties in which I consulted.

In our community support program (CSP), the approach to treating chronically mentally ill patients evolved from more traditional outpatient visits. All of us observed that chronically mentally ill patients needed more structure, more direction, and more assertive follow-up than traditional outpatient treatment offered. We also realized that patients with chronic schizophrenia do not generalize well from information given in the clinic about their living difficulties in the community. We scheduled appointments so that we could see several patients in their residences in a block of time to do whatever was required to maintain their outpatient status. The initial funding came from some of the indirect services of the clinic budget; later, it was formalized in the contract with the public funding agency, the county. After a couple of years, the state began to support CSP directly, and it was easier to find CSP staff who were even more aggressive about keeping patients out of the hospital. Transportation problems occasionally arose in our rural area. Most people in our area have some type of system, such as extended family or neighbors who help, if they do not have a car. This is necessary in a rural area. We developed a list of volunteers living in the various parts of the county who were faithful and usually available. If none of the above worked, a CSP worker would transport as needed.

Because we were committed to CSP, we never tried to develop psychiatric inpatient services in the county. We developed contacts with the two hospitals in LaCrosse with general psychiatric units, and I worked to maintain good communication and relations with the staff psychiatrists. The county also contracted for group homes, substance abuse detoxification and treatment centers, and specialty programs for problems such as eating disorders or long-term treatment of children. In general, we believed that hospitals and special living programs were needed only for the period of protection; most of the time we could develop a treatment program for specific patients in their home communities.

To those of us at the clinics, the CSP seemed to evolve just by using the resources available. It was not something we set out to create, but it did gain some national recognition. Because of my rural experience, I could be part of a national training program for CSP. This was professionally gratifying and surprised me; I certainly had not expected such an opportunity when moving to a rural area. However, I think it is a consequence of the flexibility that is common in smaller systems and rural areas.

A significant absence in a rural practice is daily contact with other psychiatrists and the frequent exposure to the results of their reading and thoughts, as well as the availability of consultation. This problem, like many in rural areas, was solvable with a little effort—the measures just were not already in place. Through my observations that people rarely practice in settings in which they do not have experience and that there are not enough psychiatrists in rural Wisconsin, it seemed important to lure psychiatry residents to rural areas.

The residency program in Madison was very receptive to establishing a rural rotation as an elective for fourth-year residents. Those residents who chose to come to work in the clinic in Vernon County were awarded a grant for transportation costs. We established a program in which the resident would travel to the clinic 1 day per week for 6 months, a realistic reflection of usual practice in rural counties. The program met my needs for increased contact with faculty and residents, and I believe it helped mentally ill patients in the rural areas of the state. All of the residents felt so good about the experience that they stayed 1 year, and all have part or all of their practices in a rural county!

Putting My Practice in Perspective

Another positive outcome for my professional growth that resulted from this program was the opportunity to take a "sabbatical." After 7 years in Vernon County, working in the same area since residency, I felt a need to work in another setting for at least a short time. One of the residents agreed to cover my practice for a year, if I found something that I wanted to do.

I had always wanted to live and work in Alaska, and I believed that the rural/frontier experience would complement my experience. I moved to Fairbanks and worked in the community mental health center for 16 months. It was a tremendous experience for my family and greatly broadened my knowledge base.

On a personal level, the year in Alaska was difficult for me and my wife because my daughter became seriously ill, and she and my wife were in California for several months for treatment. I made the trip back and forth several times, and it was exhausting to try to be with my family while maintaining my practice in Fairbanks. Many of the experiences in Alaska as a family were wonderful, but we decided to return to the Midwest to be closer to our extended families and further specialty medical care if it became necessary.

The experience clarified dramatically one of the most negative aspects of rural practice—the distance from specialty medical care. On our return to Wisconsin, we also experienced what we believe is one of the most positive aspects of living in a rural community. We felt so strongly cared for by our friends, neighbors, colleagues, and patients, that it is difficult to imagine belonging more in any other setting. Despite being gone for more than a year, within 3 weeks we felt as though we had only taken a short vacation.

Establishing a Rural Private Practice

On return to Vernon County, I resumed my half-time consulting to the clinic, but I was unsure about recontracting with adjacent counties. Before leaving the county, I had helped the clinic and the CSP program survive severe budget cut attempts, and on return, I was uncomfortable being too financially dependent on the public sector. I began gathering information and opinions concerning the viability of private practice in a town of 3,500 and a business attachment area of 15,000 to 20,000. The consensus was quite negative in terms of the financial viability. The problem was our 30-minute proximity to LaCrosse, a community with 10 psychiatrists in private practice, and well-established patterns of people in our area going to LaCrosse for all specialty care.

However, I was quite sure that seeing a different population of patients with diverse diagnostic issues would only be possible by working in the private sector. I believed that if my psychotherapy skills were not maintained or further developed, I would lose them. I had always treated a few psychotherapy patients, usually those whose therapists were uncomfortable with their medical problems. I enjoyed using those skills and the psychopharmacology skills used regularly in the public sector.

Fortuitously, a private psychotherapy group in LaCrosse asked me to be their psychiatric consultant, and I accepted. I would provide therapy supervision as well as psychiatric evaluation and treatment of their patients. As I had hoped, I learned as much as I taught, and I continue to enjoy that relationship.

My decision to leave the clinic and start a private practice came abruptly at one staff meeting. The administrator presented the state's and county's proposed budget cuts for the coming biennium. Similar to our response to previous budget cuts, she described our responsibilities to minimize the cuts and to recruit community support for our programs. I decided, "I'm not going through this again."

My wife was very nervous about the prospect, but was willing to accept the consequences, good or bad. We tightened our belt, and I started a full-time private practice. The one consulting day in La-

Crosse was stable income, and my wife would finish graduate work within a year. We would manage somehow.

The number of people who have elected to receive treatment at a private practice in our rural county is beyond anyone's guess. My schedule was full within 3 months. Many people with minimal resources selected a private psychiatrist group because of their antipathy to government assistance. Patients were unwilling to receive treatment at a mental health clinic that received government funds. This surprised me, but I realized that it results from the well-recognized independent character of most people in rural areas. Our catchment area is much larger than I thought. People regularly drive an hour or more for appointments, and 15%–20% of the practice is from LaCrosse! Most patients from LaCrosse work in one of the two hospitals or their outreach programs and want private care outside of either system. Currently, we do not even meet all the private needs in the area. Three part-time psychotherapists now work in the practice. Each of us has limited our practice, and we have constant pressure to limit our work so we do not become overwhelmed. We initially accepted Medicaid and Medicare, but found that the reimbursement did not cover expenses and give the provider reasonable compensation. Each of us allows about one-fifth of our time to patients with that insurance coverage.

I was surprised at the number of people in our rural area interested in and willing to commit to psychotherapy. Most patients present with acute histories of anxiety or panic, depression, posttraumatic stress disorder, or eating disorders, and after initial management with medication, choose to continue with psychotherapy. The practice has grown to the extent that I am now associated with three masters' level therapists who each work 12 to 20 hours per week in our office and to whom I refer much of the psychotherapy. About 40% of my time is spent in 1-hour sessions of regular psychotherapy. Slightly more than half is individual, and the rest are couples and families.

Issues of Practice Management

Reimbursement

Reimbursement for therapy is primarily from health insurance. All policies written in Wisconsin have a $2,000 annual mental health benefit that can be used for diagnosis, medication management, and psychotherapy. Most policies have a 20% copayment, but the range is 10%–50%. Many patients continue beyond the annual benefit, and a significant number of our patients were in preferred provider organizations (PPOs) or health maintenance organizations (HMOs), but were unhappy with the care. Usually their copayment is considerably greater out of plan, but they get some coverage from their insurance.

Managed Care

At present, managed care companies oversee about one-half of all patients' therapy to some degree; it is somewhat greater for therapy provided by masters' degree therapists than for care provided by a psychiatrist. We try to talk in person to reviewers and be symptom focused concerning need and type of therapy when obtaining treatment approval. We also encourage our patients to call managed care companies themselves when we believe benefits are being inappropriately limited.

Another aspect of my practice that is a personal bias, but very helpful when dealing with insurance companies and patients, is that I rarely do quarter-hour medication reviews. I have never believed that one can assess the side effects, physical situation, and situational factors that impact medication management in 12 to 15 minutes. As a result, I have good rapport with patients; they help in contacts with insurance companies when necessary and keep current with their portion of the fees.

Referrals

Now that I am in private practice, I continue to treat only outpatients, but refer to a wider variety of hospitals and specialty treatment programs that appear most beneficial to the patient. Because there is no other psychiatrist in the area, when I am not available, calls go to either the local emergency rooms, at which the family physicians treat a variety of problems, or to one of the psychiatric groups in LaCrosse who have been willing to cover during longer absences.

Part of our success is based on living and working in the area for a number of years and having connections with many agencies and physicians. However, that is not the sole explanation. From the beginning, the majority of patients came from word-of-mouth referral. Money spent on advertising seems wasted or of minimal benefit. Our surveys reveal that advertising is rarely mentioned as the source of information about our presence. We benefit from the extensive "grapevine," faith in one-to-one contact, and distrust of advertising, big systems, or government typical of rural communities.

Conclusion

My family and I are currently basically satisfied. We feel that we are part of a community that has accepted us through several transitions in our personal and professional lives. I have been able to be involved in several practice settings and to continue professional growth. My children may have missed some programs available in large schools, but may be better off with smaller programs, long-term friends, and greater individual recognition. My wife was able to stay home during the children's early years and then to return to school and work in recent years. We believe that our setting will allow us to determine the next direction our lives will take. We cannot hope for more than that.

Chapter 5

Multidisciplinary Group Practice

Leonard S. Goldstein, M.D.

*M*any futurists have stated that "change" has changed. Change has become more rapid in recent years. Anyone who has purchased a home or business computer system knows that rapid changes in technology have led to obsolescence within 3 to 5 years.

Nowhere is this change more evident than in the arena of health care. We are living through a revolution in health care delivery. I have never seen an industry group that has undergone a revolution such as that in health care, in which the producers or providers of the goods or services have been so unaware or uninformed about the changes. American medicine is being transformed, and behavioral services have, in many aspects, been at the forefront of this transformation. We are now confronted with a whole new array of forces that will shape the future, including cost issues, practice efficiency issues, outcome measures, patient satisfaction, service performance and customer satisfaction, vertical integration, and population-based rather than individual-based delivery systems. State, and presumably, federal initiatives are exerting tremendous pressure to reshape the structure of behavioral health care practice. Integrated systems that can be price competitive, but also capable of providing good service and successful outcomes, will be more effective.

Many people believe that these forces are accelerating the evolution of behavioral group practices, which will become increasingly central to the delivery of affordable, appropriate, and effective behavioral health services. Groups allow employers and managed care firms to benefit from "one-stop" shopping, as they form their alternative delivery systems. Groups can often be in a better position to measure outcomes, expand access, and lower the costs of behavioral health care services. Thus, in recent years we have seen the beginning of a proliferation of group practice formation. None of the above, however, led to my initial decision to start a group practice. I entered practice in late 1977, after completing my residency at Georgetown University and spending some time in the services division at the National Institute of Mental Health (NIMH). During both my residency training and at NIMH, I was involved with multidisciplinary team approaches. At NIMH, I devoted much of my time to community mental health centers and saw some of the advantages of multidisciplinary team approaches.

History and Development of a Group Practice

When I went into practice, my goal was (and remains) to provide the best possible care to patients. I believed that it was cumbersome to see a patient and try to be a "jack-of-all-trades" or to ask the patient to go to several other places to see several other practitioners specializing in the patient's problem. I also believe strongly in differential therapeutics and the need to match the patient with a clinician, so that there is both a reasonable chemistry or "fit" and a match in terms of the patient's treatment needs. Patient treatment needs could consist of family therapy, cognitive therapy, or other special treatments.

Thus, I started a small group practice with another psychiatrist. We planned to gradually add other clinicians who were well trained in fundamental psychiatric principles and who could also provide some specialized expertise to the group. The types of expertise included cognitive therapy, child and adolescent therapy, psychological testing, family therapy, psychopharmacology, and chemical dependency.

We decided to set up our group practice in an area where there was a need that was relatively underserved. Thus, we chose an area with relatively few mental health professionals that was beginning to grow in terms of population.

In the early years, we formed clinical teams that met at least weekly for peer supervision and to review new cases. Each team was multidisciplinary and included at least 1 psychiatrist. Over a period of 7 or 8 years, we grew from the initial 2 psychiatrists to a group of 12, with 3 clinical teams. We discovered that the team meetings, as well as our weekly staff meeting (which all staff attended), became a source of ideas about new services that were needed or innovative ideas about how to improve our practice. Our group now comprises approximately 25 clinicians.

"Service" has always been very important in our group. This entails service to patients as well as service to the clinicians who were members of the group. Specifically, we believed that having a "live person" answering the telephone was preferable to using an answering machine, and we instituted that policy early on. We offered centralized billing, transcription services, and medical records services to all the clinicians. We hoped to achieve economies of scale by centralizing these and other functions; it clearly has been successful. However, compared with a solo practitioner, our group practice spent considerably more money on staff salaries to perform these functions.

Development of Specialty Programs

In the early and mid 1980s, our group practice began to develop specialty programs. Our group has always had strong ties to the medical community and has been active on the medical staff at several general hospitals as well as eight private psychiatric hospitals. At a relatively early stage, we discovered that we received quite a few referrals of patients with somatic complaints, such as headache, gastrointestinal problems, and "stress-related" conditions. We formed a behavioral medicine track, which allowed us to bring together most or all of the resources we believed were necessary to address these patients' needs most effectively. These resource people included clinicians trained in the use of biofeedback and other relaxation strategies, hypnosis, cognitive-behavior therapies, and psychopharmacology.

In 1985, we also initiated a structured-intensive outpatient substance abuse program, which was primarily an evening program. The staff was composed of substance abuse counselors, a social worker, and several of the psychiatrists in the group. Both the behavioral medicine program and the chemical dependency program proved to be very successful and allowed the group practice to quite effectively manage the symptoms of many of these patients. It also led to close affiliations with facilities or programs that offered levels of care beyond what we were able to provide, including inpatient chemical dependency programs and partial hospitalization programs, in addition to our already close collaboration with inpatient psychiatric units in hospitals.

As a result of the behavioral medicine track, several clinicians in the group began to develop a specialty in the treatment of chronic pain. This led to the development of a focused inpatient pain program for people who had failed outpatient treatment.

Collaborative Relationships

Our group practice has always emphasized strong collaborative relationships with our medical colleagues, contact with other mental health professionals, and community involvement. Everyone in our group practice volunteers to give talks at local schools or civic organizations. Many of our members actively participate in professional societies, including psychiatric, psychological, social work, or chemical dependency organizations. Practitioners in our group have been officers in local medical societies and in the local psychiatric or psychological society.

Over the years, there has been an influx of professionals into our area; the level of collaboration and collegiality with other mental health professionals has declined somewhat, but the sense of competition has increased. Despite these pressures, our group has tried to maintain contact with our psychiatric colleagues and to keep abreast of new developments in psychiatry by attending continuing medical education activities, various departments of psychiatry meetings, and peer study groups.

Managed Care and Economic Issues

In recent years, the practice of medicine and psychiatry has become increasingly complicated, with vastly increased paperwork and increased difficulty in collecting money. This is largely a result of managed care contracting. In the "old days," you simply informed a patient that the treatment contract was between the physician and the patient, that he or she was responsible for paying the fee in full, and that he or she would need to seek reimbursement from their insurance company, if applicable. Of course, we offered to fill out any forms that the patient's insurance company required to obtain reimbursement.

With the advent of managed care contracting, however, the clinician is required to bill the payer first and is only entitled to collect applicable copayments from the patient. This is further complicated by the unavailability of accurate information about the copayment before one receives the "explanation of benefits" form from the payer, when payment is received for the first visit. By the time that occurs, you may have seen the patient three, four, or more times, and, if the patient has discontinued treatment, collecting copayments can be difficult. Because of the marked increase in administrative tasks in recent years, group practice or a shared billing service by solo practitioners has become much more advantageous. Nevertheless, with discounted fees and increased administrative responsibilities, most clinicians find themselves working harder to maintain their incomes.

It has been shown that markets go through predictable stages of managed care development, roughly demarcated into four basic stages—from loose affiliation and fee-for-service environment to fully managed competition with capitation and global budgets. In my studies of various markets, as well as through my own personal trials and tribulations, I have identified four stages that physicians and hospitals go through as the turbulent health care revolution unfolds in their respective area. The following four stages are similar to the stages of "death and dying," developed by Elizabeth Kubler-Ross: 1) stage 1 is denial; 2) stage 2 is anger, resentment, and bargaining; 3) stage 3 is anxiety, panic, and depression; and 4) stage 4 is acceptance and innovation.

Our approach has been to try to develop partnerships with managed care organizations that are invested in efficient and effective clinical care. In the mid 1980s, we began contracting with several managed care organizations. Over the years, we have discovered that some of the managed care organizations have been good partners, whereas other relationships have not been satisfactory.

The factors that make managed care companies good "partners" include timely payment, relative administrative ease, high volume of referrals, and fair reimbursement level. Other managed care companies, which "micromanage" providers, essentially punish groups of practitioners who have a commitment to an effective and efficient practice pattern. This also increases the practices' administrative costs and the general level of aggravation.

Turnaround time on payment varies widely among managed care companies. Some companies turn claims around within about 30 days, and others take 3 months or more to make payments. Our group basically is looking for relationships with managed care companies in which we can work together to achieve common goals such as high patient satisfaction, high-quality care, cost savings, as few administrative hassles as possible, and fair payment to all concerned.

Over the past 15 years, our treatment methods have become more focused and/or time effective, including cognitive-behavior therapies. We tend to use group therapies more, particularly for people requiring longer-term therapy for characterological problems or chronic, supportive, and/or maintenance treatment. Our group has also become much more sophisticated in the use of biological therapies and in the identification and treatment of addictive problems. Reflecting on this shift in practice pattern, I do not believe that it has been caused by managed care exclusively. It has been a result of a combination of externally brought about changes via managed care and new techniques or knowledge about therapeutic efficacy. Some managed care companies, however, continue to operate in an adversarial manner, in which the apparent agenda is to reduce access to necessary care or to assume that all providers are out to take advantage of the system.

We became curious about whether there was a difference in our practice pattern between full-fee or self-pay patients and patients whom we were seeing on a discounted fee-for-service or capitated basis. Our data system revealed that our patients' average length of stay (inpatient) and our patients' average length of treatment (outpatient) were virtually identical regardless of reimbursement type. We did discover that patients whose symptoms have certain diagnoses or who are in certain age groups tended to utilize more resources in the way of visits or length of stay, which was not surprising.

It is generally reported, at least in recent years, that practitioners in group practices tend to earn somewhat more than individuals in solo practice. This is not necessarily true for all individuals in all groups in all areas, but as a general statement, it holds true in nationwide polls. The more compelling reasons to work in a group, however, I believe have to do with quality-of-life issues. Individuals who need a high degree of autonomy and who are not inclined toward working in a team or a group environment will not be happy in a group practice. Many clinicians, however, enjoy the ready collegiality, mutual support, adaptability, collaboration, and centralized administrative services that a group can offer. Group practice cuts down on the "hassle factor" and provides clinicians with the opportunity to spend more time practicing and seeing patients. Group practitioners prefer teamwork rather than working individually. Group practice can be quite educational and exciting. Brainstorming about difficult cases often leads to new approaches or, at the very least, decreased practitioner guilt and validation that the patient has serious and difficult-to-treat problems.

Types of Groups

There are two basic kinds of groups, *cluster groups* and *true groups.* Cluster groups are loose affiliations of clinicians who keep their practices separate but share space and, perhaps, secretarial services and billing functions.

The Institute for Behavioral Healthcare was formed in 1988, and it is widely recognized as the national center of excellence for behavioral health care industry education and leadership development. In 1991, the Institute helped to establish the Council of Behavioral Group Practices and, in fact, has published a national register of behavioral group practices. The Institute and its Council of Behavioral Group Practices has defined the characteristics of behavioral group practices, as shown in Table 5–1.

A true group can also be defined in terms of the following five principles:

1. Common philosophy for a purpose.
2. Common information system (e.g., medical records, management systems, billing, and appointment scheduling).
3. Common leadership (i.e., a delegated decision-making authority).

Table 5–1. Characteristics of behavioral group practices[a]

Full economic and operational integration
Professional administration
Computerized management and information systems
Strong commitment to managed behavioral health care services
Ten or more full-time equivalent behavioral health practitioners
Psychiatrists fully integrated into practice
Cost-effective and flexible treatment programs
24-hour access
Quality assurance programs
Care management and continuity of care system

[a]As defined by the Institute for Behavioral Healthcare and Council of Behavioral Group Practices.

Thus, some form of internal management structure with a management team allows the organization to be flexible and adaptive. An open system is required in which information can flow from the bottom up and the top down in a circular fashion; however, it is impossible to run a group practice if everyone in the group must vote on every decision.

4. Common physical facility (required to deliver the collaborative team approach). Some groups may have satellite offices or multiple sites, but these sites are shared by the group as a whole.

5. Common risk (i.e., the fact that compensation formulas must be linked in part to the needs and success of the group as a whole). Thus, when the group does well, everyone does well, and when the group does not do well, everyone's compensation is impacted.

Adhering to these five principles and adopting policies and procedures to put them into effect transforms an organization from a loose affiliation or cluster group to true "grouphood."

Organizational Steps

In this section, I outline some of the organizational steps that have been required in the development of our group practice.

The organizational steps include the development of a mission statement, an organizational structure, a policies and procedures manual, a common information system, vertically integrated services, a total quality management system, outcomes measurement, and a compensation system. The mechanism for developing the mission statement must include the involvement of everyone in the organization, both clinical and support staff. Table 5–2 presents the mission statement from my group practice, the Northern Virginia Psychiatric Group, and Table 5–3 presents the mission statement from Park Nicollet Medical Center.

Organizational structure.   The organization of groups can be dictated by types of service offered or by the practice styles of its individual members. Our group practice has been committed for years to a general practice pattern that includes easy access, a multidisciplinary team approach, differential therapeutics, use of a hospital for stabilization only, integration of psychosocial and biological interven-

Table 5–2.   Northern Virginia Psychiatric Group mission statement

Northern Virginia Psychiatric Group is in business to improve our community's physical and mental health through the application of the most up-to-date knowledge, skills, and attitudes in the areas of psychiatry, psychology, and substance abuse.

We do this by

- Maintaining quality relationships with our referral sources, including our patients, other mental health professionals, nonpsychiatric physicians, health care facilities, the school system, lawyers, employee assistance programs, employer groups, and health plans and carriers.

- Providing comprehensive diagnostic evaluations so that our patients receive the appropriate treatment plan.

- Treating patients of different ages, including children, adolescents, adults, and elderly people.

- Providing different modalities, including individual, group, family, psychopharmacology, behavioral, and cognitive therapies.

- Offering specialized programs to provide focused and integrated treatment resources.

- Maintaining a highly qualified, licensed, credentialed, board-certified staff.

tions, and cost-effective focused treatment. Other services may include group therapy, eating disorders, and behavioral medicine. Individuals may have specific talents or specialties that will be reflected in the organizational structure, responsibilities, and leadership.

Ease of access is determined by several factors, including 24-hour on-call availability (in our group, both psychiatrists and nonpsychiatrists are available), as well as having a live person answering the telephone during regular business hours. Easy access also entails evening and weekend hours and the ability to schedule emergency appointments on the same day and routine appointments within 3 to 5 days.

Most of the psychiatrists in our group spend approximately one-third of their day doing intake work and consultations, and they spend the remainder of their time doing initial evaluations, medication management, and focused treatment. Many of the psychiatrists do family and group therapy and spend relatively little time in long-term psychotherapy, other than for more complicated cases.

Table 5–3.   Park Nicollet Medical Center mission statement

Our patients are our first priority.

We have a strong sense of accountability to our patients and to each other for providing outstanding care and service. We maintain our standards of excellence by active support of education, research, innovation, and professional growth for our entire staff. Furthermore, we reinforce our standards of practice by organizing as a physician-governed, professionally directed group practice. We serve complete health care needs in the Twin Cities as an integrated system of care, and our many specialists also serve Minnesota and surrounding states.

The mission of Park Nicollet Medical Center is to provide the highest quality of health care and service possible.

Standardization of policies and procedures. The development of a policies and procedures manual is time consuming and may be arduous, but it is essential for a well-functioning group. It puts in one place the procedures and policies that the group forms. A policies and procedures manual may include administrative issues, such as vacation scheduling or vacation policy; it also generally includes procedures and forms used for intakes, chart organization, chart documentation, procedures for handling clinical emergencies, and on-call procedures. Functioning as a true group requires precise procedures that each clinician can follow, which is ensured by the development and use of the policies and procedures manual.

Common information system. A common integrated information system is necessary for a group to function properly. The information system generally includes an appointment scheduling component, a billing and collection component, and a practice management component. Groups find that their system must provide a variety of information about elements such as length of stay, length of treatment, available treatment time, new patients, referral sources, revenue production, accounts receivable, and balance sheets. New systems are continually being developed, as the technology is becoming more sophisticated and the price is becoming more affordable. There is no substitute for testing various systems through demonstrations and satisfying yourself that the system is user friendly. The information system should also support outcomes measurement or outcomes management activities and patient satisfaction surveys.

Vertically integrated services. Behavioral services, along with the rest of medicine, are moving toward an emphasis on outpatient care. Group practices must develop and be part of vertically integrated systems that function across age groups and across the continuum of care. Thus, it is important to be able to see children as well as adolescent, adult, and elderly patients. It is also important to be able to offer services directly (or through affiliation), such as partial hospitalization and inpatient care, as well as intensive and routine outpatient care. This emphasis on vertically integrated systems has led some groups to entertain or enter into joint ventures or partnerships and has encouraged the development of regional networks.

The most compelling reason to try to set up services "in house" is that the practice has enough volume to support a significant portion of the start-up cost to deliver such a service. So, for example, if you have contracts to deliver substance abuse treatment through a capitated arrangement, it may be very easy to set up an outpatient rehabilitation program in house. When setting up joint venture arrangements, partnership arrangements, physician-to-physician alliances, or affiliation agreements, it may be advisable for the group to enlist the aid of consultants with expertise in the areas under consideration.

Total quality management system. True groups have total quality management systems. This involves the establishment of a continuous quality improvement process whereby everyone in the organization attempts to do things correctly the first time and devises ways to improve various aspects of the practice; one method is by taking surveys of patients, staff, and referring physicians. Continuous quality improvement includes an emphasis on learning to collaborate effectively and on improving knowledge about outcome. It has been clearly established that increasing quality reduces waste and cost. Outcomes management and outcomes data have been extensively discussed in recent years; only recently are we beginning to see actual implementation of outcomes management. Outcomes management appears to be an extra cost and an activity that is time and labor intensive in a fee-for-service system in which few economic incentives are tied to outcome. However, as payment for health care services moves increasingly into risk-sharing arenas, the need for good outcomes information will become apparent to everyone.

For example, a group medical practice that was capitated for a given population discovered that many elderly individuals had broken hips. This group practice studied the problem and discovered that the single biggest reason for the broken hips was that many of these individuals could not afford eyeglasses with the correct prescription. The group practice instituted free screenings and financial subsidies for eyeglasses and subsequently noted a 50% decline in the rate of hip fractures.

Compensation system. True groups need to link compensation to the success of the group as a whole. Older models for compensation generally were based on a percentage of collections, with "partners" getting a higher percentage of collections and "nonpartners" getting a lower percentage of collections. Many groups are now moving toward a base salary structure, with bonuses available for performance, based on either cutting overhead or increasing revenue. Some groups also have a pool of money available for bonuses, based on marketing activities or assistance in practice management. Increasingly, clinicians will be involved in risk sharing; as more of the revenue in a group practice becomes based on risk-sharing models, the compensation of the individuals in the group will be largely dictated by those models.

Many clinicians who have been involved in risk-sharing activities report that they have fared economically as well or better in that environment compared with a fee-for-service environment. This is somewhat reassuring. In fact, our experience has been that it is possible to practice in a clinically successful and effective way and still be reimbursed fairly.

We have not been immune to the general economic pressures on psychotherapy, however. We have maintained market share, but, at best, we are working harder for less money. Capitation contracts that may have been initially profitable have been ratcheted down to the point at which it becomes increasingly difficult to continue participation in them. The best argument to get involved in risk sharing is that your future survival will be significantly compromised if you are not experienced and capable in risk sharing.

Future Directions

It has been and will continue to be for the foreseeable future emotionally difficult for many of us who take great pride in our work and want to do the best for the patient, yet have to adapt to population-based care and alternative delivery systems. At this point, the only certainty in my life is to expect uncertainty for the foreseeable future; however, there will also always be room in health care for excellence and good physicians.

Health care, in general, and behavioral practice will be a turbulent arena in the 1990s. My experience leads me to believe that a multidisciplinary group practice will help provide support as well as the ability to thrive in the new and emerging health care delivery system.

Suggested Readings

Goldstein LS: Quality assurance and utilization review in psychiatry, in Quality Assurance and Utilization Review: Current Readings in Concept and Practice. Sarasota, FL, American Board of Quality Assurance and Utilization Review Physicians, 1987, pp 227–316

Goldstein LS: Genuine managed care in psychiatry: a proposed practice model. Gen Hosp Psychiatry 11:271–277, 1989

Goldstein LS: Pro and con: should providers accept full-risk or risk-sharing relationships with payors and benefit plans? Open Minds Newsletter, Vol 5, Issue 1, April 1992, pp 4–6

Shapiro S, Skinner E, Kessler L, et al: Utilization of health and mental health services: three epidemiological catchment area sites. Arch Gen Psychiatry 41:971–978, 1984

Shapiro S, Skinner E, Kramer M, et al: Measuring need for mental health services in a general population. Med Care 23:1033–1043, 1985

Chapter 6

Practice in a Staff-Model HMO

Otto H. Spoerl, M.D.

When I look back on the more than 23 years I have practiced psychiatry in the staff-model health maintenance organization (HMO) where I work today, I see enormous changes in the organization, in the practice style psychiatrists use, and in the role they play with other health care providers at the HMO; changes that are in magnitude comparable to the changes that have occurred in the field of psychiatry and in the health care field in general in the United States. Yet I can also see that certain features of my work here, which initially attracted me to this setting, have remained remarkably stable and continue to set psychiatric practice in an HMO apart from other practice patterns.

What Is a Staff-Model HMO?

An HMO provides comprehensive health services on a prepaid basis to its subscribers in accordance with a schedule of benefits and limitations. If it is a nonprofit organization, any excess of dues and other income over expenses incurred in providing its contractual services— the "margin"—is invested in facilities, equipment, and personnel resources. In a staff-model HMO, salaried staff provide most of the health care it offers to subscribers.

HMOs have received very mixed reviews in the publications sponsored by organized medicine (Jellinek and Nurcombe 1993; Sharfstein 1990). The American Psychiatric Association has instituted "Managed Care Hotline" on the front page of its publication, *Psychiatric News,* in which psychiatrists are invited to report their problems with managed care. Many of the reported problems have been associated with utilization and claims review processes in HMOs that use independent practitioners rather than salaried staff. However, the issue of appropriate ways to control costs is a very active topic of discussion within our own and other HMOs. HMOs throughout the country are currently in a state of considerable flux—appearances, disappearances, and changes in structure—caused by economic pressures and increased competition.

Joining the Group Health Mental Health Service in the 1970s

After having taught and practiced with an emphasis on psychiatric inpatient work in an academic setting for several years, in 1970 I was looking for an opportunity to shift to an outpatient setting. I wanted to work with patients with a wider variety of psychiatric problems, not just the most severe ones, and with patients from diverse socioeconomic backgrounds. Two major paths were open then for psychiatrists interested in outpatient work. Establishment of a successful private practice seemed to require a group of rather affluent patients and an emphasis on longer-term therapy. However, in my perspective, the "cutting edge" in psychotherapy, particularly on the West Coast, was in newer, shorter forms of therapy. The other career path involved the then emerging field of community psychiatry, but some of the looming problems were funding shortages, the necessity to become involved in largely political struggles, and increasing uncertainty over the role of the psychiatrist in that movement.

A fairly small, but well-reputed and long-established private, non-profit local prepaid health care organization was expanding its mental health service to be able to offer a new short-term mental health benefit to all its members. I decided to accept the challenge to help the organization implement this change. I found the mental health service at Group Health Cooperative (GHC) a democratically run service, staffed by a well-trained multidisciplinary team open to new ideas such as brief and very brief therapy (Spoerl 1975), easy access to mental health services (by allowing patients to self-refer), and, even then, a rather large and diverse group therapy program (Spoerl 1974). Because psychiatrists joined an already well-established medical staff organization, stability and financial security seemed to be available without the need for staff members to become too heavily involved in the medicopolitical process.

Structure and Functioning of a Modern Mental Health Service in a Staff-Model HMO

GHC of Puget Sound, the HMO I joined in 1970, is a much larger and different organization today. It has spread from the shores of Puget Sound to offer services throughout Washington State (of importance for large employers); its membership has grown to 483,000, and it is now the seventh oldest, eighteenth largest HMO in the United States. A private, not-for-profit organization with 1992 revenues of $854,000,000, it is run jointly by an elected consumer board—a team of professional managers headed by a chief executive officer and a self-governing medical staff (1,007 physicians or 763 full-time equivalents). The medical staff also manages a very large external delivery system. This consists of a panel of "preferred providers" and community professionals (and hospitals) whose credentials have been evaluated by the organization, with whom the staff contracts for specialized services according to a mutually agreed on fee schedule for services not provided by GHC.

The members of the cooperative—individuals and families who join after health screening—remain an important enrollee group and form the voting group on important health care issues. However, the vast majority of GHC subscribers now enroll through contracts offered to them and their families—without health screening—by their employers. Although many different benefits are now available, most contracts provide for comprehensive coordinated medical care, inpatient and outpatient services, and medications, with no or small copayments or deductibles. On enrollment, subscribers choose or are assigned to the panel of a board-certified family physician who acts as the patient's primary care physician in charge of coordinating his or her medical care.

The organization has recently implemented the principles of total quality management (TQM) throughout the cooperative. This movement, brought back to the United States from Japan after it was introduced there predominantly by American industry experts, aims at continual improvement of the quality of products and services through self-managed work teams, research, and emphasis on giving the customer exactly what he or she wants. The organization's governance is still that of a cooperative, with members having input on how the organization is run at all levels through voting at the annual meeting and, more importantly, through consumer involvement by membership on most of the important committees. However, over the years, there has been an unmistakable culture change from a democratically run cooperative to an organization that models itself more on structures and principles seen in efficiently run large corporations. This change, necessitated by striving for greater efficiency in view of the much increased competition in the managed health care field, has been accompanied by the involvement of increasing numbers of professionally trained managers in the administration of the organization.

Virtually all subscribers now have a basic mental health benefit, which covers up to 20 outpatient visits (with a small copayment), either self-referred or by referral from other providers, and 20 subsequent visits at 50% copayment (at prevailing community rates) per calendar year, plus a 10-day psychiatric inpatient benefit with a 20% copayment. Such benefit design obviously encourages early intervention, and indeed we find that our patients as a group are at the psychologically healthier end of the spectrum, with only small percentages presenting with severe psychiatric disorders. Our current psychiatric inpatient benefit of only 10 days per year for most members is obviously too short to fully cover many psychiatric hospitalizations. The average length of hospitalization in our system is about 12 days. However, our rate of psychiatric hospitalization—1.78 admissions per year per 1,000 enrollees or 22.9 hospital days per 1,000 enrollees—is considerably below that of most staff-model HMOs. This low figure may be attributable in part to the fact that the inpatient benefit, limited as it may be compared with coverage in most East Coast plans, is still a rather new benefit for GHC subscribers. Another factor is undoubtedly the intensive efforts on the part of staff members to utilize inpatient care only as a last resort. Considerable efforts are underway to extend the inpatient coverage in our system, but the in current market situation, the necessary dues increases are unacceptable to consumers and employers. Some of our members are covered for much longer periods under the Medicare system, and for others who require longer inpatient stays, family members, or, if all other resources are exhausted, the state welfare system may contribute funds.

Lower copayments for group therapy sessions encourage the use of this cost-effective treatment modality. Psychotropic medication coverage is the same as for other medications. "Medication checks" (i.e., 30-minute checkback appointments with psychiatrists or nurses) are not counted against this benefit, and neither is participation in a crisis-resolution-oriented "acute care group," which meets twice per week and is aimed at avoiding psychiatric hospitalization and facilitating psychiatric aftercare. These "free" services are tailored for the heavy utilizers, patients with major psychiatric disorders. They are perhaps an initial step in our design toward a two-tier benefit, one for the psychologically healthier segment and additional benefits for patients with major psychiatric disorders—a benefit design being used at some HMOs such as the Harvard Community Health Plan. The average patient coming into the mental health service is seen between three and four sessions per episode of illness. Although the service has a large free-standing outpatient clinic in downtown Seattle, a number of smaller clinics in the suburban/rural service area offer mental health services and are usually located within or close to primary health care clinics.

The mental health service has undergone extensive restructuring in recent years. The administration of the mental health services was centralized to coordinate comparable and consistent program development in the various GHC regions, so that consumers in different service areas with the same benefit could expect similar clinical offerings. A separate mental health service budget was created, featuring integration of the medical staff budget (salaries) and the operations budgets (non-medical staff and support staff salaries, supplies), thereby allowing more flexible allocation of resources to various professional disciplines. The establishment of an organization-wide centralized mental health administration also allowed successful advocacy for expanded mental health benefits and better coordination between benefit design and sufficient allocation of staffing resources. In alignment with other departments, in recent years there have been definite changes in the management style of the mental health services. Instead of electing its chief internally as in the past, the current chief was appointed by a committee, with annual performance evaluations, including feedback from the ever-widening matrix of "customers" (in TQM terms, these include not only patients, but therapists, primary care and specialty care providers, and many other people in the organization). To an increasing degree, fiscal responsibility—both for the internal delivery system and for the external delivery system described earlier in this section—is carried by the mental health administration, which, in turn, delegates it to regional chiefs and midlevel managers. In this way, each small clinical unit shares the fiscal responsibility of remaining within established budgets and has a vital, direct stake in maintaining costs.

Psychiatric Practice at Group Health Cooperative

What is a typical week like for an HMO psychiatrist? First, at GHC, full-time psychiatrists schedule themselves for a 40-hour work week with somewhat flexible hours. Some psychiatrists work 1 evening per week to accommodate their patients or a therapy group, and then they may be able to take off an afternoon during the week. Seventy percent of the 40 hours is devoted to "direct patient care" (i.e., intakes, checkback visits, medication checks, groups, and hospital consultations); the remaining 30% of the time is for team meetings, staff meetings, conferences, record keeping, clinical teaching, and telephone calls. Full-time psychiatrists in our central region currently schedule themselves for one general intake and two "special intakes" per week. For general intakes, the psychiatrist functions as a "generic therapist" on his or her interdisciplinary team and has the opportunity to work with patients with the full spectrum of mental health problems; "special intakes" are reserved for patients requiring the special expertise of the psychiatrist, such as patients recently discharged from a psychiatric hospital needing follow-up care, patients working with non-HMO therapists who are requesting a psychopharmacological consultation, or patients with complex problems referred by GHC primary care physicians and other GHC physicians for a psychiatric consultation. Psychiatrists also participate in at least two on-call systems. In one, the psychiatrists of two regions cover nights and weekends. Each psychiatrist is on call 4 weeks per year, available through a beeper to take emergent patient calls, to consult with other on-call providers, and to evaluate emergencies on site in either GHC hospital emergency room. Each mental health service also has a "doctor-of-the-day" on-call schedule so that emergency consultation is available to other therapists and nurses during clinic hours. Most psychiatrists also perform on-site consultations in the GHC hospitals or, occasionally, in nursing homes.

Because GHC does not currently operate a psychiatric inpatient service, patients are referred to contract hospitals. In two of the regions, the contract hospital is University of Washington Hospital, where a GHC psychiatric liaison nurse is stationed to provide continuity of care and a smooth transition between various levels of intensity of care.

The psychiatrist spends a large part of his or her time as a member of various teams. First, there is the area medical clinic team, a rather large, multidisciplinary team that provides mental health services for patients from one or more area medical centers. Peer consultation primarily occurs on this team for difficult cases and problematic treatment decisions. Although each clinician ultimately decides how to handle each case, the team provides feedback and helps to sharpen the focus. Another important team for the psychiatrist is the M.D./R.N. team. This team of nurses and psychiatrists meets daily to discuss acutely and chronically ill psychiatric patients on medication. There are also various specialty teams such as family/child or couples teams and ad-hoc work groups of clinicians pursuing new skills. Recent work groups have studied solution-focused brief therapy and cognitive therapy. Students and interns, from social work trainees to residents in the GHC family practice residency program, rotate through the various teams and enliven the discussion. In another region of our HMO, the psychiatrists have carved out a more specialized role for themselves, functioning essentially in a consultative role to other therapists, nurses, and other GHC physicians, but no longer treating their own patients.

There are also plenty of opportunities, but not always enough time, for special interests. If a psychiatrist has an interest in a particular clinical area or a special skill, the word spreads very quickly in our entry unit, and the referrals start to accelerate. Some of the psychiatrists regularly go to area medical centers to perform on-site consultation (see "Trends in a Fast-Changing System"); others work in subspecialty areas such as sleep disorders, child psychiatry, geriatrics, and clinical research, for which the GHC membership provides an ideal study population. (One of the central region's psychiatrists works half-time for the clinical research branch of the HMO, the Center for Health Studies.) The GHC Office of Medical Education organizes regular clinical conferences and special seminars on a wide variety of topics, and the mental health service has been featuring nationally known experts for various well-attended offerings in postgraduate education, for both GHC staff and the community. In 1993, the service sponsored a national conference on mental health issues in HMOs, in which the staff presented some experiences and innovations to a wider audience. A number of psychiatrists have clinical faculty appointments at the University of Washington and participate in teaching and resident supervision. The only form of therapy that is not generally practiced by our psychiatrists is long-term therapy, and such therapy is also excluded in the benefit. Patients who need such therapy must be referred outside, usually at their own expense.

One attraction of an HMO practice is a relatively secure and predictable income with a number of tax-free benefits, such as comprehensive medical care for the psychiatrist and his or her family (including dental care), moving allowance, life insurance, malpractice coverage, disability insurance, retirement plan, vacation, sabbaticals, paid postgraduate leave, and other optional plans such as deferred compensation and plans to pay for child care from pretax funds. At GHC, an elected committee manages compensation issues and establishes salaries using information from other HMOs and academic and private groups. The information is constantly being updated, and salaries are adjusted annually. The 1993 salary schedule for psychiatrists began at $76,000 the first year after completion of residency, reached $107,000 at the fifth-year level, and concluded with a maximum of $136,000 at the eleventh-year level (the last two figures include employer pension contribution).

Conflicts Between Patients' Needs and Coverage Limitations

Few of our patients who schedule their first appointment have read the fine print in their insurance manuals concerning restrictions for mental health coverage that apply to outpatient and, particularly, to inpatient services. Therefore, discussions about what can and cannot be provided occur frequently and form part of a working contract between the therapist and the patient. In most cases, therapy can proceed and be completed within the coverage limits, but in some situations, there is an obvious mismatch between the patient's needs—in his or her own opinion and in the therapist's best clinical judgment—and what can be provided through the organization, either by our clinicians or covered by authorized referral. The following are some examples of successful and unsuccessful cases in which I was directly or indirectly involved.

Case Examples

One of my first patients was a young housewife, whom I saw more than 20 years ago, with a syndrome featuring some very colorful dissociative symptoms mixed with anxiety and depression that responded to therapy. Treatment was successfully completed, but the patient returned several times over the years, once during a marital crisis requiring joint marital therapy, and, in recent years, I have treated her more extensively with a combination of psychopharmacological and cognitive therapy for recurrent depression. Although my treatment has never exceeded the fully or partially covered sessions per year, the therapy has clearly gone far beyond our usual "brief focal therapy" model.

A second example also involves one of my patients; a recently widowed woman in her forties with a long history of schizoaffective disorder. I have seen this patient repeatedly, often in crisis, either on our mental health service or in the area medical center where she receives her general medical care; here, she is well-known to emergency room social workers, consulting nurses, family physicians, and personnel staffing the local crisis clinic telephones. This loose network of providers, each able to provide only limited services, has enabled us to keep her out of the hospital, but the absence of covered day treatment services and scarcity of other specialized services for severely mentally ill patients have made her care difficult. After her husband, who had provided a lot of stability for her, died, her condition deteriorated, and we became very concerned about her parenting of her 12-year-old daughter. Involved in a hostile-dependent relationship with her mother, the daughter became increasingly unmanageable and began to mimic some of her mother's psychotic behavior. The daughter fortunately was covered under GHC's Medicaid contract, which provides 1 month of psychiatric inpatient coverage. After much discussion and several refusals of our suggestion to hospitalize the daughter, the mother finally agreed to hospitalization on a child psychiatry service during one of the crises. The daughter made an excellent recovery in the hospital, GHC paid in full the cost of $25,000, and the mother finally agreed to placement of her daughter into a therapeutic foster home. The daughter's development and schoolwork have improved; the mother's condition has also improved, and she will soon be participating in a social skill-building program on our mental health service.

A third case illustrates that patients with certain types of problems do not usually fare well in our system. A 16-year-old girl with anorexia nervosa whose parents are divorced was initially admitted to our contract hospital, a regular psychiatric inpatient service without special services for this disorder, because her 7-day psychiatric inpatient coverage could not be applied toward hospitalization in a special inpatient unit for patients with eating disorders. She made little progress either during or after this hospitalization, started losing weight again, and eventually was admitted to the eating disorders unit after all, with her mother somehow paying the $15,000 "down payment" required prior to admission. Her condition improved, but her mother is dissatisfied with the care her daughter received from GHC and is appealing GHC's refusal to pay for her daughter's specialized treatment.

Trends in a Fast-Changing System

As in other sectors of the health care system, the pace of change also seems to be accelerating within today's HMOs. Although GHC, for example, is one of the oldest and most stable organizations of its type, major changes in several basic aspects of its functioning are underway, which affect mental health and psychiatrists working in the system.

In order to remain in business in a market with increasingly aggressive competitors, GHC has strayed away from being just a staff-model HMO. An "options" program offers employers and subscribers increased flexibility by allowing totally free choice of providers, with a fiscal incentive to use the HMO by requiring substantial copayments for outside providers. To offer competitive premiums to employers, the cooperative reluctantly had to switch to small copayments in a number of contracts. Free-standing mental health HMOs, which provide managed mental health services to all employees at competitive rates, have approached large employers (Parker 1994). Many employers and their brokers want to avoid double-digit annual premium increases by excluding mental health benefits to lower premium rates; others wish to have more comprehensive benefits, often including employee assistance programs to increase productivity and reduce absenteeism. Employers are also concerned about easy access to the mental health system, traditionally the "Achilles heel" of HMO services, because no financial barriers exist to reduce demand for service. At GHC, the percentage of the enrolled population seen by the mental health service per calendar year has increased gradually to the current rate of 7%.

In the central region, we have made a special effort to avoid the traditional "waiting list approach" by establishing a standard waiting period of no more than 2 weeks for the initial appointment (with same-day availability for true emergencies). This results in difficult scheduling of checkback appointments. There also has been a major programmatic push for closer integration between primary care and mental health services. Because most GHC patients with psychiatric problems first turn to their family physician for help, the service has pioneered a number of initiatives to help the primary care physician assess and treat psychiatric problems. Several psychiatrists and Ph.D.-level psychologists now regularly visit area medical centers to see doctor-referred patients in brief consultation for assessment and/or psychopharmacological consultation (by the psychiatrists), with the idea that ongoing care will be provided by the primary care team. Specialized programs such as cognitive therapy–oriented brief groups for older patients with dysthymia and mild depression are also conducted at area medical centers, near the patients' homes. A senior peer counseling program offers home visits by specially trained and supervised volunteer counselors to elderly, often lonely, patients experiencing mild psychological problems. An organization-wide committee staffed by psychiatrists, family physicians, and pharmacists is developing practical guidelines for the use of psychopharmacological agents.

Role of Psychiatrists in HMOs

Ambiguity about the appropriate role of the psychiatrist in an HMO appears to be increasing. Is he or she, as in former times, the almost automatic leader of most interdisciplinary teams, or should every provider have equal influence on the team? Should the psychiatrist really be primarily a consultant, or can he or she still be the primary therapist for patients? What are the best arrangements to enable psychiatrists to be both managers and clinicians in an HMO? What mix of providers (psychiatrists, psychologists, master's-level therapists, nurses, mental health technicians, and clerical support staff) constitutes the best and most cost-effective team for a mental health service in an HMO?

Dilemmas

Some of the recurring dilemmas are associated with benefit design. How comprehensive should the basic mental health benefit be, yet at the same time, what can be sacrificed to keep the premium affordable? How much should the benefit focus on the "basically well" in the sense of educational, preventive, and health-enhancing programs in mental health and crisis intervention for life's problems; how much emphasis should be on tertiary prevention of serious psychiatric illness and associated disability? Can an HMO realistically offer a multitude of mental health benefits to be provided by a single mental health service to different subscriber groups? For example, an employer might want to negotiate and contract for long-term psychotherapy with the HMO for a certain employee group, but it could be very difficult for the typical HMO mental health service with its strong orientation toward brief therapy to set up such services.

Likely Future Developments

As mentioned earlier in this chapter, the pace of change is accelerating, and some developments seem very likely to occur in the near future. Purchasers of health care such as employer groups, brokers, and government agencies who are negotiating with our HMO have started to demand, and will probably soon achieve, greater input into benefit design and health care delivery systems. The HMO is being asked to offer an increased variety of benefits for varying population needs and preferences. Practice guidelines, not imposed by outside agencies, but developed internally; critical path diagrams assisting clinicians; and more sophisticated tools for assessment of clinical outcome will affect future care providers in all fields, including psychiatry. For example, a committee of psychiatrists, family physicians, and pharmacists at GHC recently developed a concise and much applauded practice guideline for panic disorder, and similar efforts are underway in the field of depressive disorders. Computer literacy, currently a desirable, but not required skill for physician candidates, will soon be mandatory for all GHC providers after GHC adopts a computerized medical record system.

Advantages and Problems of Psychiatric Practice in a Staff-Model HMO

The following list summarizes some of the major advantages of the modern staff-model HMO for psychiatrists starting out in practice, as well as the basic problems he or she will encounter in most such settings.

Advantages

1. HMOs offer a clinically very challenging practice with a wide variety of patients from all socioeconomic backgrounds; HMO patients are usually better educated, and the percentage of patients with serious and chronic mental illness is much smaller than in community mental health centers.
2. Patient care is to a large extent freed of economical considerations, with the benefit largely defining the limits of what can be provided; the incentives are usually appropriate for both patient and provider.
3. HMOs offer close teamwork in a stimulating setting, which provides enormous opportunity for teaching, consultation, professional growth, and close collaboration with other health care providers.
4. HMOs offer predictable income from the beginning, economic security, and a wide range of valuable tax-free benefits; limited on-call duty; predictable vacations; and sabbaticals.
5. HMOs offer excellent opportunities for psychiatrists interested in becoming medical managers, either part-time or full-time.
6. HMOs offer an ideal base of operation for the psychiatrist interested in clinical research, because of the extensive data available for its stable patient population.

Disadvantages

1. Many psychiatrists in our HMO dislike the high pressure of their practice. Their schedule never has enough appointment slots; some begin working late hours or lunch hours to accommodate emergency patients or to return urgent calls.
2. Although theoretically a psychiatrist might offer a patient more than brief focal psychotherapy, the psychiatrist's busy schedule and the constant flow of new and old patients makes longer-term psychotherapy impractical. However, the psychiatrist will certainly develop a panel of patients whom he or she will follow intermittently over the years during various crises in their lives and during exacerbations of their disorder.
3. To an increasing degree, the psychiatrist in an HMO is part of a very complex system and is involved in many matrix relationships. In order to succeed, he or she must be a good team player. This

limits his or her absolute freedom and certainly modifies the classical dyadic relationship between the psychiatrist and patient. Although the HMO psychiatrist, like his or her colleague elsewhere, works with his or her patient in the privacy of an office, the HMO psychiatrist probably is more aware of all the other subscribers waiting for an appointment and of other parts of the organization requesting his or her services. Consequently, even highly talented "solo performers" do not usually prosper in the climate of the HMO as well as good "orchestra musicians."

At last, a caveat. In this chapter, I described psychiatric practice in a particular HMO, which happens to be old, well-reputed, and financially healthy, in which a self-governing medical staff regulates medical practice. A psychiatrist considering working for any HMO should find out as much as possible about the organization. It is essential to determine the HMO's track record and reputation among local clinicians, its financial status, how the organization is operated, and whether the structure of the HMO provides the necessary freedom and support for the psychiatrist's practice.

References

Jellinek MS, Nurcombe B: Two wrongs don't make right: managed care, mental health and the marketplace. JAMA 270:1737–1739, 1993

Parker S: Warning to HMO's: improve mental health services or get "carved out." Clinical Psychiatry News 22(3):9, 1994

Sharfstein SS: Utilization management: managed or mangled psychiatric care? Am J Psychiatry 174:965–966, 1990

Spoerl OH: Treatment patterns in prepaid psychiatric care. Am J Psychiatry 131:56–59, 1974

Spoerl OH: Single session psychotherapy. Diseases of the Nervous System 36:283–285, 1975

Chapter 7

Practice on a Hospital Staff

R. Rao Gogineni, M.D.

*H*ospital psychiatry has changed in many ways since the Pennsylvania Hospital first opened its doors to admit psychiatric patients in 1750 and since Benjamin Rush, the father of American psychiatry, first became an attending psychiatrist there in 1783. The opportunities, roles, and duties of a psychiatrist in the hospital setting have changed even more dramatically over the past two decades as a result of the evolution of health care delivery systems. Many factors have influenced this change, most notably, the reduction in allocation of expenditures for state and county institutions, the increasing availability of private insurance, the burgeoning number of new freestanding psychiatric facilities, the increased power of the accrediting bodies (Joint Commission for the Accreditation of Hospital Organizations, or JCAHO) to determine standards and documentation requirements, and the increasingly litigious nature of our society and the patients we treat.

Historically, the states have assumed a major responsibility for funding and a central role in orchestrating inpatient psychiatric services (Lutterman and Hollen 1992). About 80% of the total expenditures for mental health come from the state, most of which is used to run state hospitals; in 1990, approximately $7 billion were spent on mental hospitals. Mental health, unlike other health services, has been a responsibility of the public sector, in part, because insurance coverage for individuals with mental illnesses was not introduced by commercial

The author would like to thank April Fallon for her thoughtful comments on earlier drafts of the manuscript.

carriers until the early 1950s even though general health coverage began in 1920 to 1922 (Levin 1992). Although the states still employ a significant number of inpatient psychiatrists, the number of organizations or facilities at which one can work has almost doubled in the last two decades (Redick et al. 1992). This burgeoning variety is in sharp contrast to the actual number of beds in state facilities available for patients with mental illness, which has decreased by almost one-half (Redick et al. 1992). This suggests a dramatic increase in the variety of places to work, but not in the actual number of positions available. State facilities have rather dramatically downsized their services; however, there has been a steady growth in the number of free-standing private psychiatric hospitals and general hospital psychiatric services (i.e., separate psychiatric services as part of a larger medical facility), with a concomitant increase (more than doubling) in beds available (Redick et al. 1992). Thus, although the states remain the "big spenders" for mental health care, the opportunities for employment in state and county facilities have attenuated, whereas the opportunities for employment in private psychiatric facilities and in psychiatric services of general hospitals have concomitantly increased (Lutterman and Hollen 1992).

In the private sector, when most hospitals were physician- or family-owned operations, the system often allowed considerable flexibility in psychiatric treatment and less need for meetings, rules and regulations, paperwork, and rights of various employees and patients. On the other hand, it permitted many physicians and psychiatrists to practice using antiquated and unproven treatments. As health care expanded, the rules, expectations, responsibilities, and duties of psychiatrists changed. Our role in some settings began to be more narrowly defined to include specific types (e.g., pharmacology, but not psychotherapy) or specific aspects of clinical care (e.g., individual therapy, but not family therapy).

With the advent of the JCAHO, state and federal regulations, and quality assurance and improvement programs, the psychiatrist's role was altered to incorporate active leadership in maintaining standards in the delivery of treatment. With Blue Cross/Blue Shield, commercial policies, Medicare and Medicaid, and other third-party reimbursement, the attending psychiatrist has been forced to modify treatments to adhere to third-party guidelines (e.g., decrease the treatment time of his or her patients in the hospital). As a result of mounting pressures from these reimbursement sources, the psychiatrist also has had to become acquainted with and often involved in the utilization review process, diagnosis-related group (DRG) issues, and cost containment issues. As the number of "for-profit" free-standing psychiatric hospitals increased, inpatient psychiatrists faced new challenges. On the one hand, the opportunities to practice and make a reasonable living grew tremendously. However, much to our chagrin, these hospitals frequently began to be run more like corporations, with the major goal being the production of profit rather than the mental health of patients. We became involved in the for-profit aspects of psychiatric care (i.e., making decisions based on money rather than on excellence in patient care), putting most of us in unfamiliar territory. As chief executive officers began to head institutions (instead of traditional M.D.'s), not only did the rules to judge the adequacy of patient care change, but so did the leadership role of physicians and psychiatrists.

As malpractice suits have increased, the attending physician has also become more involved in medical, legal, and ethical aspects of health care delivery. Medical ethics and the development of a more consumer-oriented medical practice have become more prominent. The need for additional documentation, justification, and general paperwork has increased exponentially.

Health maintenance organizations and preferred provider organizations have taken over a significant portion of the health care industry, further altering the role of the hospital psychiatrist. The psychiatrist often is placed under considerable pressure to adhere to a set of standards only partially determined by efficacy. For example, the pressure to shorten patients' length of stay encourages the psychiatrist to quickly introduce pharmacological interventions.

With these historical aspects as a background, I share some of my knowledge, ideas, and experiences in hospital psychiatry. I outline various aspects that I think are useful and important to an attending psychiatrist practicing in a hospital setting. I describe the results of my experience as an attending in a hospital and my observations of colleagues. For the sake of clarity and convenience, I have divided this information into various sections—opportunities, responsibilities and duties of the unit chief, medical staff composition, contracts with hospitals, how and where to look for a position, and my own personal experiential perspective.

Opportunities

The many available opportunities can be divided into five general categories: 1) university/teaching hospitals, 2) community hospitals, 3) state and county psychiatric hospitals, 4) Veteran's Administration (VA) hospitals, and 5) free-standing psychiatric hospitals. I review aspects of each of these opportunities.

University Hospitals

In a university hospital, the position often involves less direct patient care, but more overseeing of the care given by medical students and residents, providing team leadership, and serving various administrative functions. The position is generally salaried. Part of the salary comes from the medical school or other grants for teaching medical students and residents. The psychiatrist is expected to earn the other portion on his or her own by providing psychiatric treatment to inpatients, and sometimes by treating outpatients or by conducting research and procuring research grants. Most university settings have practice plans that may require one to give the university a certain percentage (20%–50%) of the monies generated in private practice (either outpatient or inpatient). The hospital generally provides benefits, including malpractice coverage, health and sometimes dental insurance, term life and some types of disability insurance, paid vacation, and paid conference time. The salary generally depends on desirability of the hospital, financial status of the institution, and academic rank. On completion of residency, the usual rank of a psychiatrist is instructor. After becoming board certified, there is often the possibility of becoming an assistant professor. The typical salary range is $70,000 to $90,000 for a beginning psychiatrist, often with the possibility of generating additional income through clinical practice or contracting with pharmaceutical companies to perform premarketing medication trials.

The advantage of a position in an academic setting for an entry-level psychiatrist is the opportunity for continued learning and growth. Psychiatrists often have access to considerable library resources, visiting lecturers with expertise in certain areas, other more senior individuals who are often experts in clinical care or on the cutting edge of particular research areas, and an atmosphere that promotes intellectual curiosity and collegiality. Of course, psychiatrists who primarily enjoy the clinical care aspects of psychiatry and do not develop expertise in a specific teaching or research area may not be well suited for this type of position, and tenure in an academic institution may be curtailed.

Community Hospitals

Community general hospitals are service-oriented medical/surgical hospitals with attached psychiatric services. The number of these services has more than doubled in the last two decades, with a corresponding increase in beds (Redick et al. 1992). They tend to be smaller than university hospitals and may or may not have teaching affiliations with university psychiatry departments. They generally have 15- to 25-bed psychiatric inpatient units, consultation services, and outpatient services. Generally, their attending psychiatry staff is composed of two to four part- or full-time psychiatrists, often with additional psychiatrists on the courtesy medical staff who admit patients to the psychiatric service. The attending psychiatrists in these hospitals generally run the inpatient service and often provide outpatient service, consultation services, and emergency room coverage. They generally conduct most of the unit chief responsibilities, as outlined later in this chapter. If the hospital has a teaching affiliation, the position will involve teaching, supervision, and training. If the hospital is located near a teaching hospital, the psychiatrist can obtain a faculty appointment to teach and supervise psychiatric residents; this enables the psychiatrist to remain in touch with academic aspects of psychiatry.

The attending psychiatrist position may be part-time or full-time. As a part-time position, psychiatrists are paid to provide general psychiatric hospital care to patients, to perform administrative duties of the ward, to attend ward rounds, to participate in utilization review and quality assurance committees, to prepare and participate in licensing and site reviews, to provide appropriate administrative and psychiatric documentation, to attend staff meetings, and to attend to emergencies (on call). In some settings, psychiatrists are salaried to provide care for a certain number of patients, but in most hospitals, you bill for your own psychiatric services (although the hospital may provide supportive billing services). For any of the other hospital services, psychiatrists may bill for the consultation they provide (psychotherapy consultation, outpatient). For a full-time position, psychiatrists may be required to perform more administrative responsibilities and/or provide some of the billable services to the hospital. The national profile of nonfederal general hospital psychiatric services is that patient billings (private insurance and self-pay) account for only approximately 35% of the revenues generated; Medicare and Medicaid account for approximately 50% of the fees (Redick et al. 1992). Psychiatrists who are completely salaried can expect the hospital to provide most of the benefits that a university setting would provide. If one is salaried for administrative time only, the hospital may provide some secretarial support, phone coverage, vacation, malpractice coverage, and health care benefits.

When all of the financial benefits are taken into consideration, the average income for a recent resident graduate tends to be higher in community general hospitals than in university hospitals, particularly after the first year or two. For the average work load, the income may be 15%–50% higher than at university hospitals, although more direct patient care and greater on-call responsibilities may be involved. In addition, one may have to sacrifice some academic interests and cope with professional isolation.

Free-Standing Psychiatric Hospitals

Because the number of free-standing private psychiatric hospitals has more than doubled in the last two decades, the number of available positions has also increased (Redick et al. 1992). Private psychiatric hospitals are either for profit or not for profit in their financial structure. The former means that investors expect to gain a profit from their investment. For the latter, any profit realized must be turned back into hospital resources or be divided among its employees. Chain hospitals such as Charter, Hospital Corporation of America (HCA), and Psychiatric Institutes of America (PIA) are examples of the for-profit variety. The attending or unit director has a similar role in both types of hospitals (see section below, "Responsibilities and Duties of the Unit Chief"). Nonprofit hospitals tend to have more courtesy staff than for-profit hospitals.

For-profit hospitals have traditionally done more marketing and referral development. The chief executive officer frequently has an M.B.A. degree and is actively involved in day-to-day financial management of units; this can be a mixed blessing for the unit director. The financial arrangement and benefit package is usually similar to the one described for a community hospital. Most often, the free-standing hospitals employ psychiatrists on a part-time basis to perform administrative unit–management responsibilities, including ward rounds, treatment team meetings, discharge planning, staff development, and marketing activities. They provide health benefits, paid vacation and conference times, and other customary benefits. The psychiatrists do their own billing for providing psychiatric service to inpatients and outpatients. The inpatient and outpatient practices feed each other. The average income in these hospitals for normal work hours is likely to be somewhat higher than in community hospitals because, on average, over 62% of the financial resources are brought in by patient fees, with Medicaid, Medicare, and other federal funding contributing a total of about 27%. Most psychiatrists who choose to work in this setting work long hours providing direct service to patients; their incomes reflect these extensive hours and may be as much as double those of physicians in university hospital positions.

Because most of these hospitals have 75 to 200 inpatients and patients in partial hospital programs and outpatient programs, they can create many specialty programs, such as those for treatment of addictions, women, adolescents, children, eating disorders, addictive disorders, and affective disorders. When providing service exclusively to such specialty units, the psychiatrist can expect to develop expertise in treating these patients, but his or her practice may become limited to this specialty.

The teaching opportunities in these settings are comparable to those in community hospitals. The relatively large number of psychiatrists on staff (15 to 50) contributes to a collegial atmosphere. In hospitals with fewer psychiatrists, a norm of long hours, and few professional activities, there is a propensity for professional stagnation.

VA Hospitals

The VA hospitals are acute and long-term care facilities that usually have a full range of inpatient, outpatient, and emergency services. The acute hospitals are medical/surgical hospitals with an attached psychiatric service. These facilities generally have a close affiliation with teaching institutions. Most of the attending psychiatrists have active teaching positions with medical schools. Over the past two decades, the number of VA hospitals has increased from 110 to 125. However, the available psychiatric beds have decreased by more than one-half (26 to 11 per 100,000 population), while the actual number of admissions has slightly increased (Redick et al. 1992). These statistics suggest that these positions are relatively stable and that major changes in the structuring of these positions will be less dramatic in the short term than in the private and nonfederal public sectors. These hospitals are generally located in urban communities. The long-term facilities, generally in suburban and rural areas, often have many hundreds of beds and various specialized and subspecialized services. Some of the long-term facilities may also have affiliations with medical schools and universities.

VA facilities tend to conduct a significant amount of research on various acute and long-term aspects of psychiatry. The role and duties of the psychiatrist vary depending on the type of facility, whether the facility is affiliated with a medical school, and the structure of the hospital. The duties are often similar to those described for university hospital settings. All such jobs are salaried. VA salaries tend to be higher than university hospital salaries. However, psychiatrists cannot establish a private practice on or off the premises. In the past, these hospitals offered excellent medical benefits (including reimbursement for psychoanalysis until the early 1980s) and very good retirement benefits. The rest of the benefits are similar to those of other salaried positions.

VA hospitals are not subject to the scrutiny of the many accrediting agencies, such as JCAHO, and other bureaucratic inspections; however, the VA has its own bureaucracy. Considerably more leeway is available for treatment of inpatients in terms of length of stay; it is an advantage to be able to discharge a patient when you believe that he or she is ready rather than because a paraprofessional from an insurance company utilization review board refuses to pay for additional days. The distinct disadvantage of treating patients at VA hospitals is that, by definition, all patients are veterans, mostly men with a relatively narrow range of psychopathology. Psychiatrists who gain much satisfaction from developing and refining new programs may find the VA system petrified in its national bureaucratic structure. On the other hand, psychiatrists who enjoy teaching, having a university affiliation, working from 9:00 A.M. to 5:00 P.M. with few weekend and on-call responsibilities, and having job security may prefer the attending position in a VA hospital.

State and County Psychiatric Hospitals

According to 1986 statistics, the number of available beds in state and county facilities has decreased approximately four-fold over the last two decades (Levin 1992; Redick et al. 1992). Yet, the percentage of patients at state and county hospitals (59%) still far exceeds those at other inpatient sites (10% private, 8% VA, 20% nonfederal general hospitals). Thus, even though the number of full-time psychiatrists has decreased over the last two decades, state and county facilities still provide ample opportunity for those interested. (However, it is likely that continued financial pressures will force administrators to find ways to maintain these patients in the community and further diminish the inpatient state facilities.)

A position at a state facility is very similar to one at a VA hospital in terms of the benefits, job security, and circumscribed working hours. However, the wealth of the program and the institution is almost exclusively dependent on the generosity of the state, and quite a range exists among states in this regard. For example, in 1990, Wyoming spent 96% of its total budget on mental health services, whereas New York spent 3.6% on mental health services (see Lutterman and Hollen 1992 for a complete review of state expenditures for mental health). Similar to a VA setting, the state and county facilities' jobs do not include weekend or night hours. Regulations prohibit opportunities for practice on the grounds of the state hospital, although unlike the VA system, practice on your own time is permitted. Many state facilities have perpetual inspections and administrative requirements as demanded by the state bureaucracies, which can be tiresome for individuals who wish to spend their time primarily with patients. The role of a psychiatrist in a state facility has little flexibility in terms of functions, and a narrow range of psychopathology is seen—most patients in state facilities have very chronic psychopathology.

Responsibilities and Duties of the Unit Chief

The unit chief/unit director/medical director of a service or ward is generally responsible for the planning, development, organization, direction, and evaluation of the clinical services of the unit; establishment and implementation of the scope of the treatment program; and coordination of all the medical services. Psychiatric administrators have the critical task of improving clinical care for patients in a complex health care environment that increasingly emphasizes cost-effectiveness and program performance. They are expected to be good managers, to embrace new, more business-oriented management methods and organizational goals, and to control the use of resources. The specific duties and responsibilities include

• Being the principal liaison between unit and other medical services
• Being responsible for the daily operation of the service
• Ensuring that each patient has the opportunity to participate in the treatment program
• Being cognizant of utilization review functions and processes and communicating problems to a utilization review administrator or physician
• Supervising and coordinating the activities of all clinical personnel, including social service workers, nurses, adjunctive therapists, and psychologists
• Developing unit goals and objectives that integrate with the hospital's mission statement
• Providing an annual/ongoing report of significant clinical issues, programs, and recommendations involving all aspects of clinical care
• Providing continuous education and in-service training to staff
• Establishing the required mechanism for the coordination and cooperation between the service's program and other hospital programs and personnel
• Communicating all policies and procedures to the service staff
• Being available to resolve management problems and patient care around-the-clock on an "on-call basis"
• Chairing treatment team meetings
• Attending patients' court hearings
• Participating in committees established by the hospital
• Assuming responsibility for patients who are assigned to other physicians in the event of an emergency
• Maintaining and improving professional skills by attending professional conventions and societies
• Screening all prospective admissions to the unit
• Participating in the hospital referral development program

On a hospital medical staff, the psychiatrist's major role is to maintain the quality standards established by the JCAHO and to prepare for its accreditation survey. Medical staff are responsible for quality assurance activities, development of clinical indicators, monitoring of clinical data, peer review of problems, planning for improved care, and implementing hospital bylaws and procedures for granting, denying, and amending clinical privileges (Coleman and Kirven 1990). One study found that the factors in the development of a good psychiatrist/administrator—past mentorship, especially during the training years; active learning about unit administration and leadership; and personality traits—all contributed significantly (Silver et al. 1990a).

Medical Staff

The attending psychiatrist is an active member of the medical staff. The medical staff has its own set of bylaws, which, in most hospital settings, are adapted from American Medical Association standards. The delineated purposes of the medical staff organization are spelled out in the bylaws and often in the practitioner's contract. Broadly, these purposes include

- Some articulation of an effort to ensure that all patients receive quality care consistent with the dictates of the law and medical ethics
- An effort to ensure a high level of professional performance of all practitioners authorized to practice, through specification of the clinical privileges of each psychiatrist, and by ongoing review and evaluation of each staff member's performance in the hospital
- Provision of an appropriate educational setting that will maintain scientific standards and lead to continuous advancement in professional knowledge and skill
- Provision of the means and route whereby issues concerning the medical staff and hospital may be discussed by the medical staff with the various hospital administrators, medical director, and board of directors
- Development and maintenance of rules and regulations for self-government of the medical staff group

The qualifications for medical staff membership are board eligibility/certification in psychiatry or other medical specialties, license to practice in the state, evidence of adherence to ethics (which translates into no reported ethics violations and a letter from a colleague or training director attesting to adherence to ethical standards), and documentation of competence, health, and experience. Appointments and reappointments are made by the medical board. Generally, the duration of an appointment is 2 years. All staff must agree to review their work with the medical director and utilization review and quality assurance committees. All must also have malpractice insurance.

There are many categories of medical staff membership. Although most hospitals have more than one of these categories, many do not have all of them. The possible categories include active, courtesy, consulting, and honorary. Membership in any of these categories is generally limited to medical and osteopathic physicians and dentists (although in some states and hospitals other professional groups such as psychologists have been able to obtain limited medical privileges).

Active medical staff.   Membership in this group is often limited to psychiatrists who regularly admit or treat patients. Generally, active members are willing to be actively involved in all the functions and responsibilities of membership, including committee appointments and emergency procedures. They are eligible to vote, hold office, and serve on committees and are required to attend a certain number of medical staff meetings to maintain their active staff appointments.

Courtesy medical staff.   This category of membership is usually limited to those psychiatrists who occasionally admit and/or treat patients in the hospital. Generally, these members are not eligible to vote, hold office, or serve on committees and usually are not required to regularly attend medical staff meetings.

Consulting medical staff.   This category is reserved for those specialists in the various branches of medicine and psychiatrists who are usually involved in consulting to other types of services.

Honorary medical staff.   This category consists of psychiatrists who are not active in the hospital, but who are given recognition or honorary status. This category is usually reserved for psychiatrists of distinguished reputation or those who are retired from hospital practice. They are not part of the active governing body and do not have responsibilities to the hospital.

Contracts

The contract or agreement between the individual psychiatrist and the hospital is a legal document that outlines the responsibilities and duties of the psychiatrist and the reimbursements, benefits, and financial arrangements between the agency and the psychiatrist. These are usually standardized to each hospital, but they also can be individualized to take into account special needs of the psychiatrist or the hospital. The agreement specifies the duration of the contract, which is usually 1 year but can be longer. The following is the general outline of the agreement.

1. *Specification of duties and responsibilities:* There may be a clause to change, add, or delete some of the duties and responsibilities, including the nature of the on-call arrangements.
2. *Compensation:* Annual salary and bonus or incentive arrangements. Some hospitals may offer a guaranteed minimum income for the first 1 or 2 years.
3. *Paid leave:* Vacation, holiday, conference time, sick leave.
4. *Insurance:* Health coverage, disability insurance, life or term insurance, and malpractice insurance.
5. *Fees:* Payment of membership dues, conferences.
6. *Billing:* Specifies your responsibility for timely preparation of all billing documents and cooperation with the billing department and utilization review.
7. *Discharge for cause:* For reasons of malpractice, professional incompetencies, intoxication, insubordination, drug addiction, misconduct, gross negligence, loss of medical license, criminal misconduct, violation of medical ethics, etc.
8. *Noncompetition:* During the tenure of the agreement and often for a specified time (up to 1 year) after the termination of employment, some agencies prohibit the psychiatrist from working for a competing hospital or agency. They may ask you not to work for agencies within a certain radius of the hospital (generally 25 to 50 miles). Many of the free-standing or for-profit organizations use this clause.

The agreement may have many other legal ramifications that are beyond the scope of this chapter to detail. It should suffice to mention that such an agreement should be thoroughly reviewed by legal counsel with expertise in contracts before signing.

Looking for a Position

Before you begin the job search, determine your preferences for geographic location and type of community to work and live in. Think of how your long- and short-term personal and professional goals will be influenced by your immediate situation. Carefully review your priorities versus the pros and cons of working in various settings to avoid much future disappointment. Prior to interviewing, recall the advantages and disadvantages within each setting—VA, state, university, and private sector hospitals. Contemplate some of the good and bad compromises between "quality-of-care" and "bottom-line" considerations.

University teaching hospital positions have many academic growth opportunities. However, university settings often place less value on clinical competence. These positions are often less financially attractive than other clinical settings. Additionally, academic bureaucracies have certain inherent frustrations (i.e., individuals who tend to make clinical decisions are those that have superior academic rank as a result of their ability to publish or acquire research grants, not necessarily because they have expertise in clinical matters).

In the private sector, one must carefully scrutinize the "for-profit" aspects of private institutions. Over the last 3 years, for-profit private psychiatric hospitals, particularly the chain hospitals, have been subject to media scrutiny. They have been accused of insurance fraud, kickbacks, unnecessary hospitalizations, and providing inadequate treatment. They have been the subject of congressional Medicare investigations. Even though it is difficult to substantiate many of these allegations, when profit making becomes the major (or only) incentive for owning the hospital, you can expect some overzealous administrators to pay more attention to profit making than to providing patient care. One way to evaluate this when interviewing at these facilities is to try to ascertain from both administrators and other staff how much pressure administrators place on the clinician to discharge patients if, and only if, their insurance ceases to pay. One must feel comfortable with the "for-profit" aspects of providing psychiatric care and corporate type bureaucracy to enjoy working in this setting. On the other hand, private hospitals are primarily responsible for expanding the role of psychiatry for the general public, lessening psychiatric stigma, and increasing the opportunities for psychiatrists.

The first year of work after training most often influences your long-term career; therefore, it may be worth sacrificing immediate gratification (whether that be a few thousand dollars a year or a geographic location) for a greater range of future options. If your future plans are ambiguous, a university teaching position is often a good choice, because it allows you to continue to grow and learn and does not constrict your future options. It is easier to transfer from an academic position to a clinical position than the reverse. During the final year of residency or fellowship, ideas from faculty and supervisors are often useful. Talking to residents graduating 1 to 2 years before you is likewise helpful.

Of course, word of mouth is the best and most frequent way to obtain a position compatible with your goals. Aside from this route, after determining your priorities, you can concentrate on the organizations that are likely to give you the highest yield. For example, if location is important and you wish to remain in the same area where you did your training, joining the local professional organizations is a good resource. Sending your curriculum vitae with a letter to all the local hospitals at which you would like to work can be beneficial. Many clinical positions are not advertised at the national level, but can be discovered in the local Sunday newspaper. In addition, many of the major journals, such as *Journal of the American Medical Association, Psychiatric Times, Psychiatric News, Clinical Psychiatry News, American Journal of Psychiatry,* and *Journal of the American Academy of Child and Adolescent Psychiatry* advertise positions. The American Psychiatric Association placement service can be of tremendous help. If you are interested in working for a private hospital, contacting the various chain hospitals such as HCA, PIA, or Charter Medical may have a positive outcome. If you are willing to move anywhere, the various placement (headhunter) organizations, such as Mental Health Management, Comp Health, Med. Pro, National Medical Registry, Inc., Horizon Mental Health Services, Liberty Health Care, Pickering Group, and Snelling Search Medical Group, can often find you a very lucrative position.

Personal Perspective

In 1982, approximately when I completed my child psychiatry fellowship, I searched for a job/practice opportunity. I consulted many colleagues, supervisors, family members, and peers. I evaluated my personal interests, personal and financial needs, academic interests and potential, and family's wishes and needs. My major strengths and interests are in providing hospital-based clinical care. I thought that I would enjoy teaching, but I realized that my lack of research and writing interests and skills would constrict my growth in an academic setting. Therefore, I decided to take a job as an assistant director of an adolescent service at a free-standing, for-profit psychiatric hospital in Philadelphia. I was promoted to director of the service 3 years later. The institution was extremely well run and well marketed. The hospital employed well-qualified, highly credentialed psychiatrists to run the various programs. One attractive aspect of this group of psychiatrists was that many of them were my former teachers and colleagues. The hospital had approximately 150 beds, with 31 of them assigned to the adolescent service. The adolescent beds were increased to 46 after 3 years because of increased demand and successful management and marketing of the service.

As the attending psychiatrist and director of the service, I actively participated in the development and management of the service. There was an aura of excitement and challenge in starting a new program. It was very gratifying and rewarding to be part of that process. I learned that to develop a program, you must consider staffing patterns, a multidisciplinary team, the architectural design of the physical site, local, state, and federal regulations, local communities' needs, and the needs and wishes of various potential referral sources (Manoleas 1991). Designing such a program was an intense, exciting, frustrating, tiring, and very rewarding experience.

During the development process, the administration (medical as well as business) was extremely cooperative and supportive, which made it easier for us to design a program plan that was based on our collective philosophies. The hospital hired an internationally known family psychiatrist as the founding director of the service. Working with and under this person enabled me to continue my education in family therapy, an area that had been somewhat lacking in my child training experience. We formulated a systems-oriented inpatient model instead of the traditional medical model. I served on various committees, including the executive committee, ethics committee, utilization review committee, and quality assurance committee. I worked closely with the marketing department and unit personnel on marketing and referral development of the unit. This was an integral part of the job. We visited various agencies, including schools, community organizations, self-help groups, religious organizations, and other mental health organizations. We gave lectures and seminars both on and off the unit on various current and important topics such as family therapy, adolescent depression, suicide, learning disabilities, alcoholism, drug addiction, aggression, school problems, child abuse, children of alcoholics, inpatient treatment, adolescent sexuality, normal adolescent development, psychopharmacology, combining psychotherapy and psychopharmacology, and transference and countertransference.

As the director of the service, my management style is more "highly relationship oriented, somewhat task oriented," rather than "highly task oriented and somewhat relationship oriented" (Silver et al. 1990b). This style has both pros and cons. Although the advantage is that it is spontaneous and democratic rather than dictatorial, allowing the people I manage freedom to be more creative, the disadvantage is that my superiors sometimes see it as vague and insufficiently directional and productive. Over time, I cultivated a leadership style that included maintaining structure and hierarchy, being available to listen to others' ideas, feelings, and input, being flexible and open to change, and being clear and firm about my decisions.

My job was to supervise and coordinate other psychiatrists, psychologists, social workers, allied therapists, and nurses. We had regular staff meetings to discuss staff-staff interactions, staff-patient-family dynamics, and the interaction of the unit with the rest of the hospital. These meetings, although very frustrating at times, were instrumental in running a smooth operation and enabling us to provide the best possible treatment to patients and their families. The social events of the unit staff (e.g., holiday parties, birthday parties, welcome/going away celebrations, childbirth/graduation celebrations) and the staff meetings helped to create and promote a family atmosphere on the unit and contributed to high morale and low burnout of the staff. The ongoing educational inservices I arranged for the staff on various current treatment issues kept staff up-to-date with advancements in psychiatry.

Morning nursing rounds on the unit kept everybody up-to-date on patient information. Multidisciplinary treatment team meetings were instrumental in treatment and discharge planning, coordinating plans with other agencies, and helping staff to work closely and cohesively with patients and their families. As the director and attending psychiatrist, my role in rounds and meetings was to give everybody an opportunity to share information, to facilitate smooth, timely running of the meetings, and to ensure that all JCAHO and other regulation requirements were met.

The successful management of an adolescent unit is a difficult task. The nature of adolescent psychology requires that peer group phenomena, peer group pressures, rivalries, aggressive and sexual acting out, antiauthority or counter-cultural behaviors, street and gang phenomena, and addictive behaviors be confronted and dealt with in the milieu. Group transference and countertransference issues also must be addressed in the hospital milieu. As the unit chief, my job was to provide both the adolescents and staff of the unit an opportunity to cope with these issues using the milieu.

Clinically, I provided individual therapy, crisis intervention, family interventions, and pharmacological interventions. I saw most of my patients on a daily basis, offering them ways to recognize and understand their difficulties, finding possible reasons behind their presenting problems (biological, dynamic, developmental, addictive, and systemic), and helping them to find better and healthier ways to cope with their problems. Treating medical problems and ordering appropriate consultations (medical, neurologic, and endocrine) are a vital part of the job. Supervising and coordinating various other treatments including group, family, school, and allied therapies (e.g., art, music, occupational, dance, and horticulture) are also essential to patient care.

By providing outpatient therapy before admission and after discharge, I ensured continuity of treatment and generated referrals to the service, which added to my value to the institution. Providing psychopharmacological consultations to the referring nonphysician therapists' patients is rewarding because you are using a unique area of expertise and essential because the nonphysician therapists are often your biggest referral sources.

During my work at the hospital, I actively taught and supervised various professionals. I supervised psychology interns, family therapy interns, and child psychiatry fellows from the local universities during their rotations on the unit. For 3 years, our hospital was the adolescent inpatient rotation in a child and adolescent psychiatry fellowship, providing me with an opportunity to teach and supervise. I also had clinical teaching positions in the teaching hospitals; I provided supervision and taught courses on inpatient psychiatry, adolescent psychiatry, addictions, and family therapy. I was very actively involved in delivering educational lectures to referring community agencies and seminars on inpatient treatment, addictions, Satanism and cults, depression, and suicide. I participated actively in local professional organizations, including the Regional Council of Child Psychiatry and other psychiatric and family therapy associations. I also attended many professional conferences to learn and remain current.

During my years of hospital psychiatry practice, direct clinical care of patients and their families was most personally rewarding. Giving lectures and seminars, providing supervision, and teaching trainees were gratifying in that they provided fun, a challenge, and a chance to learn and relearn what I had forgotten. The ability to make significant income has also been very fulfilling. I have mixed feelings with regard to the administrative aspects of the job. It is very easy to feel victimized and angry at the administration. However, I can also usually understand their position. The statement that you feel alone at the top applies to middle management (such as a unit chief position) as well. As with top-level positions, you cannot give in to a complaining attitude, but unlike positions at the top level, you feel powerless. Dealing with bureaucracy, hospitals' rules and regulations, site visits, paperwork, and third-party reimbursement are necessary evils of the job that we must live with and accept.

References

Coleman R, Kirven L: The psychiatrist and joint commission survey. Hosp Community Psychiatry 4:412–416, 1990

Levin BL: Managed mental health care: a national perspective, in Mental Health, United States, 1992. Edited by Manderscheid RW, Sonnenschein MA. Washington, DC, U.S. Department of Health and Human Services, 1992, pp 208–219

Lutterman TC, Hollen VL: Change in state mental health agency revenues and expenditures between fiscal years 1981 and 1990, in Mental Health, United States, 1992. Edited by Manderscheid RW, Sonnenschein MA. Washington, DC, U.S. Department of Health and Human Services, 1992, pp 163–207

Manoleas P: Designing mental health facilities—an interactive process. Hosp Community Psychiatry 42:305–308, 1991

Redick RW, Witkin MJ, Atay JE, et al: Specialty mental health system characteristics, in Mental Health, United States, 1992. Edited by Manderscheid RW, Sonnenschein MA. Washington, DC, U.S. Department of Health and Human Services, 1992, pp 1–18

Silver M, Akerson L, Marcos L: Critical factors in professional development of the psychiatrist administrator. Hosp Community Psychiatry 41:71–74, 1990a

Silver M, Akerson L, Marcos L: Preferred management styles among psychiatrist administrators. Hosp Community Psychiatry 41:321–321, 1990b

Chapter 8

Practice of Child Psychiatry

Kathryn Ouzts, M.D.

I wrote this chapter to convey not only how this particular southern practice is conducted, but also how much enjoyment such a practice bestows. I discuss specific issues that arose during the evolution of my practice in the hope that they will be useful to residents making difficult decisions about which directions to choose at the conclusion of their training. My current practice has evolved over the 15 years since fellowship. If the current trends toward a different system of payment for medical care continue, private practice will change dramatically and probably in unexpected directions in the next 10 to 20 years. If there is a guiding principle, it is that flexibility and diversity serve you best in making the most of the serendipitous opportunities that present in any setting.

Description of My Current Practice

I am a child psychiatrist in outpatient private practice and the child psychiatry attending on the inpatient adolescent unit of a teaching hospital in a medical university setting. This combination offers me the opportunity to teach and to be exposed to new techniques of treatment and new theories from contact with academicians, residents, and fellows. This contact, of course, immeasurably enriches my own repertoire of treatments and allows me to observe a great variety of psychiatric illnesses as they are affected by different biological and psychotherapeutic treatments.

My practice is in Charleston, South Carolina. Currently, I spend 5 mornings per week as the clinical attending for the adolescent team on the child psychiatry inpatient unit at the Medical University of South

Carolina's Institute of Psychiatry. I then work at my adult and child psychiatry private practice in the afternoon from 1:00 or 1:30 P.M. until 6:00 to 6:30 P.M. 4 days per week (Monday through Thursday). On Friday afternoon, I catch up on administrative tasks at the hospital and the office. The outpatient department's child psychiatrists cover weekend call on the unit with us, so I am on call approximately once every 2 months, or 7 times a year. I cover for my outpatients 24 hours per day, 7 days per week, while I am in town. Five of the other child psychiatrists in private practice are willing to exchange coverage for one another when someone wants to go out of town. Emergency calls or medication calls are relatively infrequent.

General Treatment Approaches

I prefer to treat outpatients—children and adults, couples, and families—using brief or longer-term psychoanalytically and cognitively oriented psychotherapy, with medication used as an adjunct to therapy. If I have worked closely clinically with psychologists or social workers, I will diagnostically evaluate their patients for medication, but I find it difficult to monitor medication if I do not have the therapeutic relationship established in psychotherapy. Also, I find that patients resent spending the time and the extra money for an additional therapist. Therefore, they are more resistant to the idea of medication and less compliant. I will gladly provide medication follow-up for a patient I have followed initially in psychotherapy.

With respect to my outpatient practice, approximately 5% of my patients receive medication checks every 3 months, 40% (usually adults or older adolescents) receive individual insight-oriented psychotherapy, and 5% receive marital therapy. Fifty percent of my patients are children and adolescents who receive a combination of family therapy, individual psychotherapy or play therapy, and medication (approximately 75% of all the children and adolescents seen).

Occasionally, an outpatient requires hospitalization, or a patient I have supervised the treatment for on the inpatient service will follow up with me as an outpatient. Usually, however, inpatients and outpatients are two very distinct groups. Inpatients tend to be lower functioning and to seek treatment only in a crisis, whereas outpatients tend to be more psychologically oriented, higher functioning, and seek treatment before the situation becomes a crisis.

My approach to hospital care (before becoming a unit attending) included the following: individual therapy three times a week; coleading with another child psychiatrist two problem-oriented groups per week; conducting a 15- to 20-minute treatment review of each patient with a treatment team (and the patient) each week; and meeting with each family and patient for 30 minutes to 1 hour to obtain historical data, review the problems leading to admission, develop a plan to manage the major problems on an outpatient basis, and discuss medication. Family meetings, which I often conducted with the social worker, eliminated phone calls and misunderstandings about treatment and medication and, therefore, saved time in the long run.

Court-Related Evaluations

Occasionally, I perform court-related evaluations, such as those involving divorce, custody, and child sexual and physical abuse, but the dilemma is that they are time intensive for brief periods. Frequently, the evaluation must be completed in a matter of weeks, which can involve several sessions per week. If your schedule is already full, you must do the evaluation in addition to your regular hours. Also, the court hearings or trials are scheduled at the convenience of the court, often causing you to cancel the regular appointments of very responsible invested patients who resent this as an avoidable inconvenience. Your regular patients often repay you by "forgetting" the next appointment, or you consequently work longer hours to provide the canceled sessions outside of the court hours.

Collection of court charges is also difficult, because only the evaluation sessions are usually paid for in advance, despite my general policy that the court hearing or trial must be prepaid. My usual fee for court appearances is $1,000, at an estimated rate of $250/hour. Depositions cost the same amount per hour. However, payment for depositions, court hearings, and trials is unreliable, because neither party in the dispute is usually totally pleased with the psychiatric recommendations or the outcome. In addition, lawyers demand a retainer fee up front, and by the time a psychiatrist is consulted, neither party may have the money to pay this fee.

Fees are reduced by the courts in several ways. Once information from the evaluation is obtained, the lawyers can subpoena this information, although it may not be in the form of a report without calling you as an expert witness. The judge may also decrease the amount agreed on between the psychiatrist and the public defender. Frequently, the person who is least invested in the evaluation or who dislikes your findings will simply refuse to pay after the services are rendered. For all these reasons, I carefully select only three or four court-related cases each year.

The Evolution of My Practice Into a Success

To describe the process by which my particular practice evolved into a rewarding and successful enterprise, it is necessary to trace its development. After experiencing the blizzard of 1976 during my last year of a child psychiatry fellowship at Massachusetts Mental Health Center in Boston, my husband and I knew we were headed in the right direction—south. We chose Charleston because we wanted to live in the South, only 2 to 6 hours by car from our parents, on the coast, and in a small- to mid-sized city with some history and an active cultural life. We attended the first Spoleto Festival in Charleston and fell in love with it. The fact that the Medical University of South Carolina and four small colleges were also located there was an added bonus. Only later did we realize that a medical school is a mixed blessing because it constantly produces a new supply of excellent residents who wish to remain for the same reasons we selected Charleston.

The tricounty area around and including Charleston had a population of approximately 350,000, served by nine psychiatrists and no private child psychiatrists when we arrived. We wrote a letter to each psychiatrist to inquire about the practice opportunities in the area. All of these practitioners contacted us by letter or phone and were cautiously supportive. However, only one group was interested in renting us office space and in referring patients.

My husband is an adult psychiatrist, and we completed medical school and psychiatric residency at the same time. This was always a distinct advantage during training, but it became more of a liability after we completed residency. One obstacle is that psychiatric private practice communities become ambivalent about absorbing two psychiatrists simultaneously, although they are generally receptive to one new practitioner.

In starting, we had to deal with a number of issues related to practicing in a group. The first was associated with the call schedule.

The group we joined was composed of three psychiatrists and three psychologists. The psychologists could cover for outpatients only. One inpatient psychiatrist was paired with each outpatient psychiatrist or psychologist for 1-week rotations, from Monday to Monday. In that way, medication and hospital admission issues that arose on an outpatient basis when the psychologist was on call could be managed by a psychiatrist. This call arrangement worked so well in terms of sharing the work and dealing with clinical issues that when our original group split up, we all continued in the call schedule.

The second problem involved the secretaries. The original psychologist and psychiatrist who formed the group owned the office and hired the secretaries; everyone else rented office space from them. We soon learned that "he who hires and fires" receives first priority when work overload occurs. Furthermore, in this situation, we could not revamp the billing system, which was antiquated and inefficient. To cope with these problems, my husband and I hired our own part-time secretary who worked out of our house. Although this proved to be more difficult than we anticipated, we found a bright, hard-working high school senior who was highly recommended by her teacher.

As our practice grew, file space became severely limited, and this became an increasing liability that interfered with efficiency in billing, filing for insurance, and managing patient reports and records. Eventually, three of us moved out and opened our own office.

The three of us practiced in the new location for 2 years. We all became increasingly aware that we had to buy, not rent, an office for tax and business reasons. My husband and I also discovered that we preferred the simplicity, quiet, and confidentiality of an office shared just by the two of us. Most of the psychiatrists and psychologists in the area tended to buy suites of offices with the intention of renting some to defray costs. In our opinion, this approach is shortsighted, because it continually contributes to the pool of new competitors. Therefore, we decided to buy our own office, with no intention of expanding to include other mental health professionals.

Having completed part of our training in Boston, we were familiar with the idea of analysts having offices in their homes. Although I wanted the official office to be separate from my home, I wanted to retain the homelike atmosphere. Therefore, when an old 1840s farmhouse became available merely three blocks from our home, we bought it. My office contains a working (and well-used) wood-burning fireplace; it is furnished with Queen Anne wingbacked chairs, a small writing desk, an antique traveling trunk, and two child-sized Queen Anne chairs. Live plants constitute the remainder of the decorations. (I'll never forget the admonition of one of the social workers in Boston, who stated that if a therapist could not keep the plants alive in his or her office, then she had serious doubts about his or her ability to keep patients alive. Furthermore, half-dead plants are worse than no plants at all.) Watercolor paintings done by friends and former patients decorate the walls.

Adjacent to the main office is the playroom. Two ceiling-to-floor windows are a dominant feature. When the trees have leaves and a gentle breeze wafts through the open windows, you feel as though you are in a tree house. The equipment I find necessary for the playroom includes books, games, puzzles, and giant plastic containers holding Legos® and larger projects of child patients. A four-poster doll bed, which I got from Santa Claus at age 7 years, rests in one corner and has survived the depredations of many small boys and girls who insist on sitting on it. All the toys are neatly displayed on the shelves in easy reach of even the smallest child. A covered basket or two are scattered about to encourage exploration. Inflatable Barbie doll furniture (located in some unknown catalog by my mother) has been a godsend. Hyperactive oppositional boys deflate it routinely with gusto without destroying it (sometimes much to their dismay), whereas prissy, rather obsessive girls routinely inflate it and arrange it with much enjoyment during doll play. As yet, the furniture has been indestructible and invaluable in play therapy.

Perhaps the most unique feature of my practice is my "therapy hounds," a variety of mutts of assorted sizes, ages, and personality styles. They assist in "breaking the ice" with children and putting them at ease, as well as provoking associations that are therapeutically valuable. For example, one emotionally restricted 10-year-old boy was reminded of his own dog that had died several years before. He cried while describing how he could still feel the impression in the bedcovers at the foot of his bed where his dog used to snuggle up at night when he was dropping off to sleep. Parents always seem relieved when the office is so homelike and nonthreatening because they frequently seem concerned that simply coming to see a psychiatrist will be traumatic for their child. One of our dogs, I am convinced, was raised with a latency-aged boy with an attention-deficit hyperactivity disorder because, despite middle-age and a generally phlegmatic nature, she perks up, clumsily gambols around the office, pricks up her ears, and plops her feet on the counter as soon as any 7- to 10-year-old boy of this description enters the office. My secretary and I have come to respect her astute diagnostic acumen, and we prepare the office accordingly when Blackie exhibits the above pathognomonic behaviors.

Another unusual feature of our new office was the use of a computer. Although we have had a succession of more and more powerful computers, I believe that the most useful computer component was the original laptop that I still use to record my office notes. The laptop is used as a terminal on a UNIX system, not as a free-standing computer in its own right. Because it is portable, it is useful for hospital consultations or routine hospital notes. My husband wrote personalized office programs with the aid of friends in the computer field for our accounting, billing, notes, insurance, prescriptions, business and personal checking accounts, business letters, reports, forms, and paging and phone dialing. Commercially available programs can perform most of the functions accomplished by our personally created custom software.

For the computer novice, finding or developing a computer program requires an ongoing commitment and a major investment of time and money. Computerizing our office has contributed greatly to our success professionally and financially, because it has allowed us to personally do much of the secretarial work ourselves and so eliminate the expense (approximately $12,000 to $15,000 yearly) and the headaches of hiring, paying, and supervising another employee. One secretary is sufficient for our current two-person practice.

My husband thinks that he could manage his practice without a secretary as long as he has the computer with its personalized programs for scheduling, billing, and insurance claims filing. For me, it would be difficult without a secretary because of the frequent scheduling changes due to childrens' illnesses, school schedules, and extracurricular activities. It is not cost-effective for a child psychiatrist earning $90 to $100 per hour to perform secretarial services worth $8 to $9 per hour. On the other hand, when a psychiatrist is just opening an office and is uncertain of how busy he or she will be initially, not having a secretary saves money. Other benefits of not having a secretary include the patient's increased sense of confidentiality, the patient's direct contact and negotiation with the psychiatrist in every aspect of the session, which provides additional grist for the mill of therapy, and the elimination of the extra employee/employer taxes, along with their extra paperwork.

Hiring a good secretary is more difficult than you might imagine. Despite being a child psychiatrist, I have managed to choose three secretaries with various learning disabilities. All of them, however, have had a knack for relating well to my patients, both children and adults, which is of prime importance to me. They generally have the first contact with patients and referrers, and the impression they convey frequently determines whether the caller follows through with the appointment. Their job description includes scheduling, completing the physician's portion of insurance forms, billing, collections, filing, typing our organizational letters and filing information from various professional organizations, buying snacks for us and the children, shopping for office supplies, completing the quarterly tax forms, balancing the personal and business checkbooks, triaging phone calls, babysitting children accompanying adult patients, contacting and opening the door at home for servicemen making repairs, sorting the mail, mailing requested charts for former patients, and organizing and filing professional journals. Obviously, they are expected to have many talents. Benefits include money toward purchasing health insurance, a retirement plan after they work for us for 3 years, and a holiday bonus.

One of the consistent difficulties has been absenteeism when the secretary's child is ill or has special events or activities. We had assumed adolescents would generally be healthier than younger children, but this has not proven to be the case. As a child psychiatrist, I am sensitive to this issue and have tried to be a reasonable role model as an employer. However, as a small-business owner, I am increasingly aware of the liabilities of hiring a woman with children. On the positive side, a secretary who has children has experience with children at different stages of development, relates comfortably to children with problems, enjoys entertaining them when necessary, has increased sympathy and empathy with parents who have a child with a problem, and has an increased ability to coordinate schedules and to solve problems.

Because psychiatry is a time-based specialty, "no shows" are costly. The initial appointment "no shows" were dramatically decreased after we began mailing practice information sheets to potential new patients. This sheet included directions to the office, my educational background, services offered (such as individual child or adult, couple, family psychotherapy, medical evaluation, medication), the handling of insurance forms, general parameters for evaluation and therapy, telephone calls, and cancellations.

I expect payment in full for the evaluation, which consists of one session for adults and two sessions for children or adolescents. However, a deferred payment arrangement may be worked out after it is certain exactly what portion of my fee the insurance will cover. My current secretary created a payment agreement form, and she works out the details with patients after they have discussed the need for a payment deferral arrangement (which amounts to an interest-free loan) with me in the session. If they wish, the secretary prints up a series of payment blanks similar to checks, with stubs that have the specific amount owed per time period. The "check" portion is mailed with the payment to us so that the patient and the office have a serial record of payments.

Patients are expected to file their own insurance forms and to contact their insurance agent or the insurance department of their company concerning the extent of coverage. My secretary will help patients fill out their portion of the form, and we supply monthly bills and a computer-completed universal insurance form provided for a fee by the American Medical Association. The patient is responsible for mailing these with his or her portion to the insurance company.

I will not take insurance on assignment because I expect patients to pay the difference between the insurance payment and my fees. The one exception to this is Medicare. However, I only accept Medicare from patients who have retired or been placed on disability during the time I was treating them. The problems with Champus or Medicaid/Medicare are that 1) the government holds the physician criminally liable if there is a billing error, which means a fine of $2,000, and 2) keeping up with the regulations is a full-time job. The government programs' payment schedule is at least $30 to $40 below my usual fee, and they tend to pay at the end of the quarter or later. This practice unfortunately is similar to that of the insurance companies, and amounts to the insurance companies' obtaining the interest on money I have earned. The paperwork associated with these programs is also excessive and onerous. And finally, if their funds run out prematurely, they retroactively lower the hourly fee for which they originally contracted in order to accommodate their shortfall.

When I was billing for my hospital work, I did accept Champus on assignment because a significant number of patients reneged on their agreement to pay the copayment portion and the difference between the insurance payment and my fee. In addition, several parents kept the insurance money. If I had agreed to assignment and the check was accidentally mailed to the parents who cashed it and refused to pay me, then Champus was obligated to repay me directly. If I had not accepted assignment, nothing could be done except that I could write to the officer in charge of the parent's military unit about the matter, who would then pressure the offending parent to pay me. Now that I am an inpatient attending, this is no longer an issue because I am salaried.

We no longer use a collection agency for overdue bills, because their approach proved less effective than having my secretary contact patients by phone to discuss payment. In addition to the secretary's contacting the patient about the overdue bill, a series of messages of increasing sternness are automatically added to the computer-printed bill according to the number of days the bill is past due. Any payment on the bill eliminates these messages.

My collection rate has ranged from 59% during my first year in practice to an all-time high of 112% in my fourteenth year of practice. Currently, my 1993 collections are running at 90%, which is the overall average for collection rates over the 16 years of my practice. The total amount of bad debt over 16 years has been $59,300, or $3,706.25 per year, or approximately 38 therapy hours per year.

Managed Care

Up until the present, I have refused with impunity to join preferred provider organizations (PPOs) or health maintenance organizations (HMOs), but in the changed health care climate of the past 6 months, I have lost at least six "good" outpatients due to the parents' companies electing to change insurance programs and join a local PPO or HMO. In an effort to keep insurance company–sponsored PPOs and HMOs out of our community, numerous local physicians in different special-ties formed a physicians' HMO named Healthsource, with the intention of providing basic medical care at the lowest possible cost, with physi-cians monitoring the care and the costs. Although I supported the concept as the lesser of two evils, I thought that I was busy enough (having had a waiting list since my second year in practice) to risk not joining. Although I encouraged my husband to buy stock and to join to indicate our support for this proactive, realistic effort to compete with the insurance companies for clinical control, I was hopeful that the child psychiatrists would be able to negotiate a more acceptable set of criteria for the standard of care covered if they remained unified and did not immediately join. However, the Medical University of South Carolina decided that all specialties would join Healthsource and so our solid ranks were broken.

With managed competition as the favored approach for the coming health care reform, I have reconsidered my original position on HMOs and Healthsource and have joined the ranks as a Healthsource specialty physician. This means providing services covered by Healthsource at a discounted rate (10% discount for children and 4% discount for adults). A routine Healthsource insurance policy allows 20 outpatient visits per year and three 10-day hospitalizations per year. Partial hospitalization programs are paid out of hospital coverage, which translates into 20 partial hospitalization days per 10-day hospital admission. Only doctors who have signed up as providers are covered by Healthsource currently.

I suspect that a limited panel of specialists will be appointed at some point in the near future as the "vertically integrated systems" favored by health care reform are developed locally. In such a system, inpatient, partial hospital, residential care, and outpatient services would be managed and coordinated by health care organizations. For the moment, because these vertical systems have not yet been formed, it seems advisable to join every plan available to keep my personal options as open as possible. Since physicians may still choose whom they see and when they see them, I am not restricted to seeing only Healthsource patients or even to seeing them preferentially.

Selection of New Patients and Referrals

The referral source, the type of problem, the age of the patient, and my general caseload at the time are all factors in the selection of new patients. The freedom to develop office policies that suit me and to still maintain a waiting list is a function of many factors, including being in an office with my husband as the only other practitioner, having a partner whose views are in accord with mine, being the first child psychiatrist in private practice in an underserved area, and, most importantly, providing the best care I can at a moderate cost. Patients and referrers alike look for an obvious interest in and enjoyment of your work with patients. Sincere enthusiasm and an optimistic attitude inspire trust on the part of patients and referrers that you will do a good job regardless of the circumstances. Once such a reputation is established, referrals generally follow.

A wide variety of referral sources is preferable to a few, because multiple sources are most likely to provide a steady supply of new patients when openings in your schedule occur. An excess of referrals creates a no-lose situation, because nonemergency patients may elect to go on your waiting list, and emergencies may be referred to other psychiatrists with whom you then earn "credit."

A variety of activities have helped me to meet other physicians and health professionals and to become known in the community. Examples include the presentation of a case for pediatric grand rounds at the Medical University of South Carolina and joining and attending the meetings of the Charleston County Medical Society, the South Carolina Medical Association, and the American Psychiatric Association (APA; the local Coastal Chapter meetings, the state district branch meetings, and the national convention meetings). When the state district branch of the APA contained enough psychiatrists to divide into three chapters, I served as the first Coastal Chapter president, then the president-elect for the district branch, and this year as the president of the district branch (the state organization). Because of an interest in the legislative issues and my involvement locally, when the position of deputy representative to the assembly (of district branches) of the APA became vacant, I was asked to serve in this capacity. This post has provided a wonderful opportunity to meet psychiatrists from all over the country and to become aware of the similarities and differences of the problems they are addressing and also their frequently innovative and creative solutions. I have also acquired a broader perspective on major issues confronting psychiatry by participating in the thoughtful, articulate debates in the local multistate area councils and in the general assembly sessions.

Other organizations that have provided a means of meeting other potential referral sources, as well as providing moral support and education, are the South Carolina Pediatrics Association, the Charleston County Medical Society, and the Coastal Medical Society. This last society is one of the more unusual medical organizations in our area. It was founded in the 1930s in order to introduce the specialists in Charleston to the general practitioners in the outlying towns of the tricounty area, so that the general practitioners would know the doctors to whom they were referring. This group was recommended to me by the same female colleague who introduced me to the pediatricians at the Medical University of South Carolina. Professional networking is very helpful and has resulted in invitations to present grand rounds not only at the Medical University but also at other local hospitals. The presentation of talks to school parent-teacher associations, Sunday school classes, and high school health classes is another way to educate the lay public about psychiatric illness and treatment and to simultaneously advertise your practice in an inoffensive manner.

Consulting to various agencies is another useful way to stabilize your income, to make new referral contacts, and to add variety to a straight outpatient practice. For me, this involved becoming a paid psychiatric consultant for Horizon House, an alternative therapeutic school program for children and adolescents who were unmanageable even in special education classes for the emotionally handicapped. Although unpaid, serving on the board of family services of Charleston afforded me valuable experience with a local agency. Because family services is subsidized by the United Way, it can offer a sliding fee scale, which means that this agency is not directly competing for the same patient population a private practitioner would see. Serving on the board, which established the first halfway house in Charleston, was also satisfying to my husband and me. Recently, I began working one half-day (5 hours) a week at a local residential treatment center. This is particularly satisfying because it allows me to follow over a long period adolescents I have evaluated briefly during hospitalization.

Nonmedical volunteer work affords another enjoyable means of contributing to your community, meeting new friends, and also widening your contacts and your referral sources. For example, I have been an active member of the Junior League, a national organization of volunteers who establish needed programs in their communities and staff and fund the programs until they become self-supporting. It has been enjoyable to work with other bright, capable women volunteers to research and develop programs to deal with prevention of teen pregnancy or to establish a halfway house for women with alcoholism. In a similar vein, serving on the school liaison committee of the Charleston

County Medical Society, which is working on a program in the schools to test for and track teen pregnancies as a prelude to developing effective pregnancy prevention programs in this area, has been rewarding.

Problems Encountered

One of the major problems initially in practice in a small city was the lack of a psychiatric inpatient unit for either adults or children and adolescents in one of the downtown hospitals. The only child/adolescent psychiatric inpatient unit was located at the Medical University of South Carolina, and only child psychiatrists employed full-time at Medical University of South Carolina could admit directly to that unit (at that time).

In trying to grapple with this deficiency, I became involved with a for-profit hospital chain that was building a free-standing psychiatric hospital in our area. Unfortunately, the major result of this involvement was that I learned what to avoid in hospital affiliations. Although not related specifically to the practice of child psychiatry, my experiences apply to all psychiatrists who do inpatient work, and are therefore worthy of comment here.

The major issue in determining acceptability of an inpatient institution is its commitment to an adequate standard of care, rather than simply to generating the highest possible short-term income for shareholders. In contrast to traditional nonprofit community hospitals, some for-profit chains have no long-term investment in the community, but merely aim to generate high income in a short period and sell out at a profit as soon as possible.

The telltale signs of such an operation are numerous. Expenditure of large sums of money on advertising with relatively little on program development or continuing education for the staff, hiring of staff with the least possible amount of training (such as general rather than psychiatric nurses) at the lowest possible cost, substituting generic "programs" for individualized treatment, overloading the more highly trained staff with administrative responsibilities, and laying off staff whenever there is a temporary drop in the number of admissions are among the hallmarks of a profiteering administrative policy.

Admitting physicians at such an institution may find themselves in chronic conflict with administrators over admissions policy. Administrators may want to keep beds filled without regard to the appropriateness of patients for the unit or their need for acute hospitalization. In addition to fostering poor practice, this type of policy has hidden costs. The increased frequency of contested claims absorbs much staff time and energy, and attending psychiatrists find themselves rendering services for which they are not reimbursed. The divergent goals of the doctors and the administrators tend to make dialogue and collaborative solutions all but impossible. After several years of attempting to find a satisfactory way to work within such a system, I was ready to leave.

Fortunately, the chairman of the psychiatry department at the Medical University suggested that some of my colleagues and I consider admitting our private inpatients to the child/adolescent unit at the Medical University. Another male child psychiatrist and I had been supervising the child fellows' treatment of outpatients for 2 years. We leapt at the chance and agreed to admit our inpatients to the Institute of Psychiatry for 1 year, at the end of which we would each have the option of being the attendings on different teams rather than treating patients directly ourselves.

At the Institute of Psychiatry, I have been very satisfied with the staff, staffing patterns, staff benefits, unit programs, quality and performance of the residents and fellows, and the responsiveness of the administration to clinical needs. Because the job of attending has consumed 12 to 15 hours per week in addition to the 20 hours for which I originally contracted, the hourly pay is significantly less than the amount earned per hour in my outpatient practice. However, hidden costs always lower the hourly rate on an outpatient basis as well. For example, phone calls and letters to patients, teachers, other physicians, divorced parents, employers, agencies, and insurance companies or managed care companies consume much additional time over and above the hour spent with the patient. Also, although interesting and essential, continuing medical education is expensive and time consuming whether pursued via seminar courses and/or books and journals. However, because I wish to financially support my outpatient office from my private practice, it has been necessary to maintain approximately 18 to 20 hours of outpatient treatment. Therefore, the work week is approximately 60 to 70 hours (excluding continuing medical education). One of the benefits of working at the Medical University is that physicians can attend any of the continuing education seminars free of charge.

Conclusion

With this, I conclude the summary of my personal odyssey into private practice. As is the wont of adventures, the circumstances change, and it is the quick wit of the protagonist in problem solving that wins the day. Surviving the challenges is its own reward. Private practice currently encompasses many arrangements. Practitioners who can preserve their individuality while pooling their business resources will be better able to mount rapid and adaptive responses to change. Despite the frustrations, private practice has been challenging and rewarding overall, and I highly recommend it.

Chapter 9

Psychoanalytic Practice

Harvey L. Rich, M.D.

*T*hroughout its entire century-long history, psychoanalysis has attracted and sought people who are scholarly individualists. If I were to describe myself, I would admit to a love of art, scholarship, and personal and professional individualism. I make no apologies for my science and firmly believe that it will survive and thrive for years to come. Psychoanalysis is still the best methodology available to investigate and treat deeply buried psychological symptoms.

When I think of a succinct way to tell someone how to start a psychoanalytic practice, I am reminded of two well-worn quotes: Franklin Roosevelt's "The only thing we have to fear is fear itself," and John Kennedy's "Ask not what your country can do for you, but what you can do for your country." This may sound corny, but using these principles is how I began a practice, and it is how anyone else can. The quotations embody the basic idea of this chapter. Prepare yourself, prepare yourself, prepare yourself. Become the best prepared clinician in whatever area you choose. Avoid the generic title of your profession (psychiatrist, psychologist, social worker, nurse practitioner) and the eclectic label. Be somebody special in a poorly standardized field. The public cares for quality and will recognize it and reward you.

Twenty years ago, starting up a practice was not very different than it is today. I did not start my professional life with a psychoanalytic practice because I had to first support my training. That meant my personal analysis, my institute tuition, and my supervision. All were full fee and out of pocket, with no third-party assistance. That part is easier now than it was before. But I have jumped ahead of myself.

Background

Let me go back to the beginning. Who am I, and how did I end up with a "psychoanalytic practice"? What was my professional interest and personal philosophy that guided me in this direction? My initial interests were in the fine arts and liberal arts. However, I also had a mother who told me I had to be a doctor—so I became a doctor. My sense of the world is spacial and tactile, even in the way I have studied great literature. When I read, I create "form and texture pictures" of what is written. I hear visually and "see" word concepts in their spacial and tactile relationships and tensions.

Once I gave up my dream of being a sculptor, I was prepared to become a surgeon. Having been a surgical technician had shown me that the aspects of anatomy, technique, and equipment suited me. Then one day, while doing a summer clerkship in a city hospital's psychiatric ward, I listened to an analyst interview a young male patient. I was awestruck. I knew that I could do that, and I believed that I could do it better than the doctor I was observing. When I look back on that moment, I believe I was struck by the power of the interviewing process. The interviewer had a power—by dint of his theoretical model—that allowed him to move into the recesses of his patient's mind and slowly uncover the pathology. It was surgical. It was mesmerizing. I knew that I had to gain that skill, that power.

I then began to take electives in psychiatry, which in those days were largely taught by psychoanalysts. Their grasp of the human mind was vast, intricate, powerful, and highly useful. It did not take long for badly suffering people to be relieved of their symptoms. That was a surprise. It was not what one heard in the press or in the jokes on television. I also noticed that those teachers who had the psychoanalytic training were indeed superior in treating patients than those without. My wife noticed that they were also more content with their professional lives and more interesting people. To me, the advantage of psychoanalytic training was inescapable.

Training

I did not jump into it though. It was as daunting in those days as it is now. The training analysis was out of pocket and full fee. Unlike now, when insurance contracts cover training and nontraining analyses to the same extent, no insurance was allowed, because it was a "training analysis" and not a clinical necessity. The time commitment was significant. The requirements for graduation were 4 years of classes, four supervised analyses with one to termination, and a personal analysis, which did not have to reach termination before graduation. My wife finally had the courage to put into words what I was thinking. I had to begin my training because I would never be satisfied offering my patients, and my own image of myself, partial treatment. If I had become a surgeon, I would not have stopped at general surgery. I reasoned that I might as well do psychoanalytic training while I was relatively "young" and my children were young.

The training took me 5½ years. In general, it was wonderful fun. Not all my classes were stellar—our teachers were not professional teachers, but volunteer analyst teachers—but the depth of study into the mental processes was very satisfying. I remembered how at the end of the second year of medical school, I had a feeling of total mastery of the anatomy, physiology, and chemistry of the human body. I knew how they all related to each other and could marvel at the complexity of this natural creation. That is how psychoanalytic training felt toward its completion. I understood how the human mind, greater than the sum of the human brain, could be understood and treated.

I believe that our new colleagues have been very misguided to believe that deep and thorough treatment is not practical or effective and would not be well received by patients or, more important, by third-party payers. They are no longer exposed to the analytic teachers in nearly the personally continuous way we were then. That is a pity. The experience I have just described is difficult to replicate today. When I go to a training program and show how an analyst works, it both impresses and depresses the same group. The latter effect is because the young residents do not know or understand how they will acquire this skill if they want it. It frequently seems to them to be beyond their reach.

One of the things that analytic training did for me was to enable me to speak to the patient's deepest psychic structure or character. This is impressive in its depth and truly imparts the sense of real potential of the talking cure. Such ability cannot be faked. If I had one thing to attribute to the success of my practice, it is the real depth of understanding that my training has afforded me.

My Practice

I have achieved a practice that suits me quite well. I see approximately 57 to 63 hours of patients and supervisees a week. That breaks down to nine patients in four-times-weekly psychoanalysis, 4 hours of supervision, and the remainder psychotherapy, mostly more than once weekly. I will see some patients only once weekly while awaiting more time to open for greater frequency of treatment. I teach at the Washington Psychoanalytic Institute and am active in local and national professional groups. My office is at home, which has allowed me to spend time with my children, and lets me be in close proximity to my avocation, woodworking. I believe that my practice is larger than that of most of my psychoanalytic colleagues. Many have practices of 40 hours, with two or three psychoanalytic cases and the rest psychoanalytic psychotherapy, some with and without medication. Having worked to become a supervising and training analyst helps a bit, but not as much as most people would think. In general, I am willing to work more hours, but also, like only a few of us, the majority of my referrals are for long-term intensive psychotherapy or psychoanalysis. I have pondered why this is so, and have arrived at different answers over the years.

I seem to have greater success in moving a patient from the consultation phase to the working alliance. I do believe that my attention to a careful, detailed consultation and my conviction in the efficacy of this treatment method are a large part of how I have been able to build such a stable referral pattern and how I can get patients to agree to do the work. There are a few of us whose practices look very much alike, and in each one of us you can see the same conviction and dedication to prepare ourselves for focusing on this major method. I have not sought eclecticism. I have instead sought a great depth of experience and supervision in psychoanalysis. I have further communicated that focus and depth to my professional and public communities through my public speaking and writing.

A friend of mine who is trained in psychoanalysis recently moved to a middle-sized city in the Midwest. On arrival, he was the only psychiatrist who could do in-depth psychotherapy, let alone psychoanalysis. Instead of melting into the "standard of practice for the community," he boldly asserted his expertise to the professional community and the public. He tells of how one day he got a call from a psychiatric colleague who said that he had a patient who had refused his medications and wanted to "talk." "Talk?," said the psychiatrist, "Talk? . . . well, there is a guy in town who talks!" He made the referral to my friend.

Patient Characteristics

My patients are generally neurotic or characterologically disturbed up to the mild borderline level. I do not see severe borderline or psychotic patients, mostly because I do not do hospital work or extensive psychopharmacological treatment. My work is exclusively psychodynamic. When medications are indicated, I ask a skilled colleague to administer and follow the drug treatment. This is personally desirable, optimal for the patient, and optimal for the psychoanalytic treatment method.

My true interest is in the patient's mind. I am intrigued by the newest discoveries about the brain and, most particularly, what they imply about the workings of the mind. Psychoanalytic training, starting with Freud, a neurologist, has always focused on how the brain of a given person is affected by years of childhood dependency and cognitive and psychic development. In general, I keep up with these recent discoveries, but not at the detailed level of a colleague devoted to neurophysiology and psychopharmacology.

I love to carefully uncover unconscious processes which, by definition, are not apparent to the patient. I never tire of watching the patient master these processes and integrate the power of the unconscious, rather than be its hapless victim. I get very "involved" with my patients. Whether they are in psychoanalytic psychotherapy or psychoanalysis, I see them often. I get to know them better than they ever knew themselves and surely better than anyone else before knew them. The process is intimate and difficult. It is complicated because, in my style of practice, I do not hide behind the method. It is vulnerable because my use of my own personality as a tool for cure leads to narcissistic exposure. It is most gratifying to see the process work, to see me use myself in a precise manner, and to bring about structural change in the mind of a patient. I seek all of this in my practice.

I also am a person who likes results. It would not be satisfactory for me to see someone for a long period without a direction of improvement being evident. This does not mean that I get impatient with the slow, obsessional patient who does not color the room with affect and free-flowing verbal pictures. Improvement is both an interpsychic and intrapsychic factor. The intrapsychic changes are frequently subtle to the observer, but they are of major impact to the overall psychic harmony of the patient. As I said before, it was a surprise to see how quickly symptom relief can be achieved with the talking treatments. Such changes are most satisfying to me as well as to the patient. People like to heal themselves, without exchanging dependency on unconscious forces for chemical forces. This does not rule out the appropriate use of medications, but it does change one's clinical judgment about them. Patients are frequently grateful for the relief brought about by the use of medications, but beyond that, they appreciate the power to cure themselves on a deep level and to gain control of a large area of mental life they never knew before. It is this collaboration that I seek and find in my practice.

Setting

I also seek a certain kind of setting for my work life. I have never been a person who needs great institutions behind me or uniforms on me to make me feel genuine. I do, however, need an aesthetic setting. Few hospitals or doctors' office buildings meet these requirements. My office is more like a living space. When privacy is available, I will even supervise a candidate from the Institute in my garden. I have found that this factor of setting is most important to me. I believe that one aesthetic enhances another, as one soul enhances another. This is most important when dealing with the deepest unconscious affects and conflicts of another person.

Starting and Establishing a Practice

Starting a practice is very difficult today. It really was not so different when I started out 20 years ago. The chairman of the psychiatry department in which I had done my residency spoke clearly and darkly when I called to ask his advice regarding private practice versus his invitation to join the department. I wanted him to say, "Sure, Harvey, set up your practice and I'll send you patients to fill your hours." Instead, he spoke of the death of private practice and the future of medicine being University-centered. His words burned into my dreams of being a private practitioner and creating my vocation just to suit me. His clear and threatening tone also haunted me in my dreams: "Go off on your own and you'll be on your own and get nothing from us." That is exactly what happened. In 20 years, I have not received one referral from my beloved alma mater. As I look back, that was all right; I might not have made it on my own with their help. I was forced to invent the wheel for myself, and now I know that that process, in and of itself, is what has culminated into a successful practice.

So, what about Franklin Roosevelt and John Kennedy? I was scared to death. I refused my fear and used it to energize me. My first patient was referred to me by a patient I had seen in my residency. After 6 hours, she told me she was going to be seeing a senior colleague, an analyst, who she had been seeing without telling me. Another referral came in the nick of time, but there was no flood of calls. Thinking of "what we could do for others," I began an enterprise of speaking to any group about anything they wanted to hear. As a result, I became a member of the "medical advisory boards" of several helping groups, such as the Childbirth Education Association. A few referrals came from each of these interventions—many were "bad" referrals, but a few were "good."

I then began to practice my golden rule: never refuse a referral. That includes self-referral or colleague referral. A corollary of that rule is to accommodate everyone. For the first few years, I saw patients whenever they needed to be seen. I only turned down rare requests. I believe that during those first years, the most important aspect of building a successful practice was to create a sufficient number of satisfied patients who have completed their treatment to act as a "critical mass" of referral sources. Your fellow colleagues will not do it for you. If you have the choice to nurture your colleagues or your community, choose the latter.

Early in my practice, this policy meant seeing some patients who were more disturbed than those I currently treat. On occasion, this even necessitated using psychotropic medication, but usually I was able to manage such patients' symptoms with more frequent sessions and/or more supportive therapeutic measures. Even today, I rarely refuse a request to see a patient for evaluation, although I refer many more of them to a network of trusted colleagues that I have built up.

Currently, like two decades ago, it requires 5 to 10 years of very hard work to build a psychoanalytic practice. In that time, you can generate many referral sources and build up that "critical mass" of satisfied patients who will think of you when someone recognizes their special maturity and asks how they came by it. Only a few referrals per year are necessary to maintain a psychoanalytic practice.

My next rule is to offer a complete consultation. Once I have established a diagnosis, I present the patient with a thorough discussion of his or her problems, underlying character structure, and the resultant strengths and weaknesses related to treatment. I then make an honest and direct treatment recommendation, without any hyperbole. Arriving at this might take three or four visits. Beforehand, I would have told the patient that it would take that much time for me to say something intelligent and that I would strive to do so once I had a clear picture of the problem for which they were seeking treatment.

It is tempting to put aside one's best judgment to keep a patient who is, for whatever reason, desirable. I do not believe that patients should determine their treatment plan. If they want to control the treatment frequency or modality, do not agree to treat them—a treatment started on such footing is doomed. Worse, you will have compromised your professional integrity in both your eyes and the patient's. This type of debasement can only frighten a patient at the unconscious level (if not consciously) and end your alliance then or in the near future. I have now had many experiences with patients who did not initially accept my recommendation, but came back later for this very reason of professional integrity.

It is a fair question to ask if a person starting out today can operate the same way I did, and still do, when setting up a psychoanalytic practice. I believe that it is more difficult today, only because there are more detractors and competitors "out there" who will try to dissuade a patient from psychoanalytic treatment. A person starting out now is often not of the same conviction that I had when I began. This combination is damaging and must be overcome; 1 or 2 years should be allowed for that. After overcoming these obstacles, the rest is very similar.

As a supervising analyst, I have been able to observe the people starting out. Some just take to it, and their practices are filled when I try to refer to them. Others limp along, unable to get people into treatment or keep them in treatment. Usually, this is not an economic issue, but, again, one of identity, conviction, and hard work. I have had a young colleague whose practice was very unstable refuse a referral because some time element or fee issue was, as they said, "just not convenient." Those who succeed are often the ones giving lectures through our Psychoanalytic Foundation and teaching in our extension programs for the professional community.

Financial Issues

Today's antipsychotherapeutic climate has affected us all. Quite simply, psychoanalytic practices have benefited by being excluded, in large part, from the third-party payment system. My patients are not poor, but they are not all necessarily rich either. In general, they are middle to upper-middle class economically, and the cost of treatment is very much felt in their budgets. It is now a regular part of the consultation process to evaluate the patient's capacity to pay for treatment. I openly discuss financial arrangements with my patients. Sometimes we use financial statements and even accountants' advice to come to a plan of action regarding financing the treatment. I do not expect the patient to make all of the compromises. I will do everything from delaying payment on part of the bill to reducing my fee in order to avoid any interference in the treatment by third parties. I would say that about 10%–20% of my practice is based on some such creative financial arrangement.

Of course, this process is loaded with psychological information and meaning in the treatment setting. As the saying goes, "It's all grist for the mill." I have found that patients can understand and appreciate devotion to their privacy, as well as the importance of not placing future obstacles in the way of treatment. Recently, when a "managed care" office required telephone permission for every two visits, I told the patient that this would be incompatible with my solo practice and his interests. We talked it over, during which time I offered to help him find a therapist who would be able to handle such interference. He called back later that day with a creative solution he had worked out with his employer. His policy allowed for him to avoid all managed care interference if he were willing to accept only 25% reimbursement. His employer was willing to create a medical fund for him using before-tax dollars to pay for the rest of the bill. Because he was in the 40% bracket of combined federal and state taxes, he ended up with a 65% copayment arrangement—15% better than his managed care option would offer.

Affording psychoanalysis is more a matter of mind than it is of money for many people. There is no question that treatment is expensive, but the real obstacle is helping a patient recognize both the need and the advantage of in-depth work. If you say that treatment will cost $20,000 annually and sit back silently, I would be surprised, and even a bit concerned, if the patient rushed into the deal. However, if you do the consultation, ending with a thorough discussion of the patient's pathology, underlying character structure, and treatment options, along with a primary treatment recommendation, the path is far more laid down. The patient will still react to the money issue, but now it is in a proper context, and it means the beginning of an alliance. Financial matters can be put into perspective, as in the cost of not treating, relative to other commitments, such as tuition. Believe it or not, patients can understand that they need and can benefit from such a financial commitment when it is properly laid out for them.

I also am very careful about the patient's confidentiality in dealing with any third-party payer. I will write careful, nonrevealing narrative summaries to third-party payers, but I use the utmost discretion regarding the patient's confidentiality. This is true even when the patient gives me written permission to correspond with a third party. The bottom line for me is that I would rather earn a little less money or delay my earnings and still have a practice filled with interesting patients who can benefit from my treatment, than cooperate with an unjust system.

Professional Organizations and Colleagues

I should mention the role of the Psychoanalytic Society and Institute in my professional life. First, I must also add that the Psychoanalytic Foundation, the part of our local organization that interacts with the professional and public communities, is a major focus of my work. I currently serve as its president and chairman of the board. It is purely voluntary for all the clinicians who work through it, but the rewards are real and plentiful. We teach psychoanalytic psychotherapy, run a low-fee clinic, and teach a wide range of short courses aimed at professionals and the public. The exposure provided by the Foundation is definitely helpful to my practice in terms of informing others about who I am and what I do clinically.

The Society and Institute provide my major professional circle and a major part of my social circle. I like many of my colleagues personally. They are bright, articulate, socially interesting, and caring people. Society and Institute contacts with colleagues of all levels of training represent the main source of referrals from within the profession. The Society and Institute also are the main arenas of my postgraduate education and intellectual challenge.

For many years, the institutes and societies of the American Psychoanalytic Association seemed to work hard to gain the reputation of rigid orthodoxy. I have to say as loudly as I can, "THAT HAS CHANGED!" Today, there are many changes in theoretical and clinical thinking and administrative policy of institutes and societies. There is an atmosphere of embracing new people and ideas, while still holding to the best and most essential parts of traditional psychoanalysis. I find that my contacts at the national level, which in recent years have increased rapidly, are the most gratifying in my professional life. There are wonderful, exceptionally smart and stimulating people around the country whom I speak to regularly on the telephone and see at least twice yearly at meetings. They have great influence on my life professionally and personally. The loneliness of the clinician that we all talk about in private practice is gone from my professional life since I have become active on the local and national levels. These people also become familiar with me on a personal level, which then allows them to make careful referrals to me; in recent years, I have noticed that more of my referrals come from out of town. However, that was never my motive for national or local involvement; I would not give up such contact for anything.

The greatest pleasure for me has been that I have evolved in my own identity as a clinician to include practitioners of all academic backgrounds as colleagues. I consider a well-trained psychologist or social worker as my colleague. Psychiatry let the field of psychotherapy go, and other fine people have picked it up. I choose to be part of any group of colleagues who value the unconscious and the structures of mental processes in their clinical work.

I recognize the value other "psychotherapies" can have. I simply do not practice them. Remember, I do not believe in being eclectic. However, that does not mean I choose to remain ignorant. I do try to remain current by reading journals and books. Time constraints do not permit much more.

Conclusion

I believe that I have the best of several worlds. I can work, with a full practice, in a style that suits me. I do not turn my back on patients, but I do not abide unjust interference either. I enjoy the respect and collaboration of psychiatric colleagues and those well-trained colleagues from other disciplines. I teach, supervise, write, and lecture. I am very active in local and national psychoanalytic organizations, and the company of those colleagues is most fulfilling. I earn a very good living with very low overhead. Many people—planners, managers, and even other psychiatrists—want to put psychoanalysts like me out of business, but patients do not. How long can this last? I do not know. If government regulation will simply leave me out of the system they need to develop to deliver a baseline of health care to the people, I will survive.

In the end, my psychoanalytic training, including my personal analysis, has made me a much better clinician, regardless of the depth of psychotherapy I administer. It has also provided me with the knowledge base that allows me to maintain a full practice. It keeps me calm in the face of regulatory panic and, most importantly, focused on my patients' needs.

Chapter 10

Practice of Psychopharmacology

Kenneth Piotrowski, M.D.

*T*he challenges of going into psychiatric practice are different today than they were 20 years ago. The uncertainties about future care delivery and funding make all physicians uncomfortable but are especially confounding to the new professional psychiatric care provider and business owner. Almost a quarter of a century ago, I was fortunate to choose a psychiatric residency training program that was medically oriented. This firm foundation allowed me to evolve a private psychiatric practice concentrating on psychiatric diagnosis and psychopharmacological intervention. In the early years, I also provided individual, couple, family, and group psychotherapy, but my true interests were always in the biological arena.

I decided to go into private practice after my second son was born with Down's syndrome. Prior to that time, like most residents, I was evaluating the pros and cons of different types of practice. The challenges of being on the faculty of a university program seemed exciting and stimulating. The rewards of regular hours at a salaried position with a governmental mental health facility were appealing. However, being in business for myself was the only avenue that offered the hopes of maintaining the income I would need to provide security for my son. At the same time, this has come at the price of working very long hours that might otherwise have been spent with family. In recent years, I have taken more advantage of my freedom to adjust my work schedule without checking with an employer. I can go to as many or as few continuing education courses as I feel is appropriate. Although I am not a millionaire, I have continued to earn a reasonable income for the hours I choose to work.

Choosing and Starting a Practice

I was ambivalent and anxious about starting the practice. After I finished my training, I had the opportunity to join an established psychiatrist with a large practice in an area that was psychiatrically underserved. My wife's family was in the area. It would have been an easy and comfortable transition. The area itself, however, was industrial, and the climate left a lot to be desired. When I pointed out that we would be able to afford to take many vacations to nice places, my wife astutely replied that we could choose to live in a place where other people took their vacations. This observation was difficult to argue with. Although the anticipated problems of starting a practice in an unfamiliar area led to many sleepless nights, we decided to give it a try. There were many psychiatrists in the particular resort area on the west coast of Florida that we chose. However, several of the established psychiatrists seemed to be quite busy working what I considered to be a regular work schedule. Other established psychiatrists felt that there was not enough to go around. A "black cloud" speech followed inquiries about a new psychiatrist making a living. With much trepidation, I jumped into the world of private practice.

Eli Robins, then the chairman of the department of psychiatry at Washington University Medical School in St. Louis, either sensing that the departing residents had some trepidation, or as part of the fatherly advice he gave to all his departing residents each year, told us that we would be successful if we saw patients in a timely manner. He defined "timely manner" as within 24 hours. This turned out to be very good advice. Shortly after arriving in town, I realized that only one other psychiatrist was providing this service. That psychiatrist was exceedingly busy and not at all threatened by new psychiatrists coming into town.

Many of the psychiatrists seemed to work 9:00 A.M. to 5:00 P.M., Monday through Friday. I decided to offer expanded hours. The patients who did not want to take time off from work were grateful. Referral sources seemed somewhat surprised but were happy to get their patients in quickly. During the first 2 years of my practice, I had evening office hours 4 days a week and Saturday mornings.

Regular office hours did not start until 1:00 P.M. In the mornings I worked in the hospital doing consultations and seeing inpatients. On Monday, Tuesday, Wednesday, and Thursday, I saw patients from

1:00 P.M. until 9:00 P.M. in the office. I did not make a formal announcement regarding the extended office hours. When a referring physician's secretary or nurse called my office to schedule an appointment, he or she was frequently surprised to discover that the patient could be seen at 8:00 that evening. This quickly got the attention of referral sources. To keep the office staffed in the morning to respond to referral sources and to assist me in the afternoon and evening, full- and part-time secretaries were required. This schedule proved to be very successful in terms of building a practice, but was physically and mentally demanding. My family life suffered, but the practice steadily grew.

The Start of Change

Toward the end of my second year of practice, I was treating a dysthymic female patient with limited communication skills and low self-esteem. Consciousness-raising groups were very popular at the time. I suggested that my patient start to participate in these programs. The patient responded well, and soon I began referring additional patients to other consciousness-raising groups in the area. However, within a relatively short period, a leader of one of the groups called to inform me that the last several people I had referred to the program were "too sick." They were "depressing" other members of the group. I solved this problem by hiring the leader of a consciousness-raising group to conduct the group in my office. This was my first experience in private practice of not doing everything myself. This led to the development of more focus groups. Eventually, I introduced more traditional psychotherapy groups by hiring allied mental health professionals who I paid an hourly fee.

After group therapy sessions, I noticed many of the patients seemed to enjoy "hanging around" and interacting with one another on a social level. Because the office schedule was rather tight, this practice became somewhat burdensome. Yet it was clear to me that this postgroup socialization was very beneficial for many of the patients.

A small apartment above my office became available for rent. I thought this apartment could provide space and atmosphere, not only for additional groups, but for socialization after the groups. I had hoped that the increased overhead would be made up by starting additional therapy groups. I was wrong. My solo practice did not generate enough patients to form enough additional groups to cover the added expenses.

The apartment was rented on a month-to-month basis. After 4 months, I gave up the apartment. In retrospect, a group of psychiatrists could have generated more patients to start more groups. This also might have been an opportunity to start a day treatment program. Twenty years ago, a day treatment program did not exist in my area. One of the reasons it did not exist was that there did not seem to be any insurance coverage for outpatient day treatment programs.

Hiring Allied Mental Health Professionals

After seeing the utility of working with allied mental health professionals in group therapy, the next step was to expand and hire them to work with patients on an individual basis. I started with a part-time psychiatric social worker. This led to associating with a psychologist. By referring patients for counseling and psychotherapy, I was able to concentrate on my primary interests of evaluation and medication management. The number of allied mental health professionals grew. Within 3 years, the professional staff comprised one psychiatrist (myself), two full-time Ph.D. psychologists, three full-time psychiatric social workers, and a part-time psychiatric nurse. The allied mental health professionals also received direct referrals from other sources besides myself. I was always available for advice and consultation. Supervision of and consultation with allied mental health professionals consisted primarily of assistance in making a psychiatric diagnosis and discussions about which disorders could be expected to respond to somatic intervention. They were experienced psychotherapists, and I did not believe that I had much to offer them in that area. However, only after working with them for a while did I really feel comfortable in knowing that they could and would refer patients appropriate for somatic intervention back to me.

In addition to time requirements, it seemed as if there was never enough space available. The clerical staff was present from 8:00 A.M. to 9:30 P.M., Monday through Friday. Some mental health professionals shared offices (i.e., a few would work only during the days, and others would work in the late afternoons and evenings). This was not a very satisfactory relationship, and each full-time therapist really did need his or her own office.

Each therapist had an area of special interest and expertise, and this allowed me to match the type of patient to the type of therapist.

However, providing support and psychiatric backup for this many people proved to be quite burdensome. Although I did not keep track of the number of extra hours or patients I saw, I found myself working an extra hour or two almost every day. I needed another psychiatrist to join me.

Financial arrangements with allied mental health professionals varied over time. In the early years, they were either independent contractors or salaried employees. The independent contractors chose their own hours and set their own fees. They were given a choice of either being paid a percentage of the gross collected or a flat hourly fee. This model was patterned after the same compensation system used in real estate offices and beauty parlors. Each signed an independent contract agreement. This document clearly identified them as responsible for paying their own withholding taxes and providing their own malpractice and workers' compensation insurance. They were not eligible for any employment benefits. Another group was hired as regular contract employees. In this case, I set the hours and assigned the type of work to be done. The full-time salaried contract employees were given benefits such as paid vacations and health insurance. At times, an allied mental health professional chose to switch from being a salaried contract employee to an independent contractor. Interestingly, this always led to a great increase in productivity. A course given in the mid-1970s at a meeting of the American Psychiatric Association on running group practices identified these compensation models. In the mid-1980s, articles started appearing about the uncertainty of using independent contractors. At present, the allied mental health professionals I work with are independent practitioners who set their own hours, collect their own fees, and pay a fee based on actual office overhead for shared expenses. When there were many independent contractors keeping their own office hours, therapy rooms were difficult to schedule. The obvious solution was to expand.

Every time we expanded to gain additional space, we attempted to "finally get enough space," but soon all the office space was filled again. Management was not my forte. Two attempts with business consultants did not seem to work much better. After spending a day or two in the office, they made suggestions for more efficient use of resources. However, within a short period, it became clear that the changes they suggested led to different problems. It appeared that the issues of running a multidisciplinary psychiatric practice were specific enough that even business consultants who have dealt with other types of medical practice were not much help. In the end, our own process of trial and error seemed to work out best.

Forming a Professional Partnership

Fortunately, a well-trained psychiatrist who had been in private practice in New York City for several years was visiting the area and contacted me. He had already decided to move to the area and had heard that I needed an associate. I felt very comfortable with him from our initial meeting. His style of practice was different in that he preferred psychotherapy, but he was knowledgeable about the kind of work I did. After many discussions about what we each wanted in a practice, we put our understandings of how things should proceed on paper. We both wrote down as many things that we could think of. We reviewed articles in *Medical Economics* on partnerships. There was no other psychiatric group in town at the time, so I talked to colleagues in medical and surgical groups to find out what worked for them, what mistakes they had made, and what things they would do differently. In the end, we decided that compatibility was the main issue and did not try to anticipate every contingency. We agreed to an informal arrangement that paid a fee toward overhead with the understanding that if we both still liked each other after a year we would become equal owners of the practice. If this were not the case, my potential partner would leave and start his own practice. I did not think restrictive covenants were fair or enforceable and so decided not to try to use any. At worst, I would have had a little extra office space with resulting increased overhead for a period of time. Fortunately, things worked out well, and we became equal owners of the business a few months earlier than scheduled.

As some allied mental health professionals left to go into their own solo practices, new ones joined us, as did a third psychiatrist. My partner and I worked well together. His interests were more in the area of individual psychotherapy, and he was also quite competent in providing consultation and supervision to other mental health professionals. The third new psychiatrist enjoyed both individual psychotherapy and medication management.

For personal reasons that had nothing to do with the practice, my partner decided to leave. The partnership, which was in the form of a corporation, was dissolved, and we stayed together for a period of time in an overhead-sharing arrangement. It became clear to me during this time that I did not want to continue worrying about the number of hours I had to work and being responsible for the supervision of and consultation to all the allied mental health professionals in the office. The timing seemed to be fortuitous because my 10-year lease was just about up. The lease was extended for 1 year while we all made individual plans to pursue our practices on a solo basis.

Forming an Overhead-Sharing Partnership

Paradoxically, I ended up associating with another psychiatrist and clinical psychologist who were in the process of opening an office about 5 minutes from where I lived. The structure of this new practice was very different. It was not a professional partnership or corporate entity, but an overhead-sharing partnership. Although corporate practice structures were common when I started, I had not found enough advantages to make this extra trouble worthwhile. For example, the corporation might provide personal protection from general negligence, but not for malpractice suits. In the partnership, I do not have any responsibilities for supervision. Because one of the overhead-sharing partners functions as the office manager, I do not have any administrative responsibilities. My sole obligation in the partnership agreement is to write out a check at the end of each month for one-third of the overhead expenses for the duration of the lease of the office space.

This transition allowed me to reevaluate the type of practice that I wanted to conduct. After 19 years of a very hectic pace, I decided to decrease my patient load and make time for new pursuits. One of the pursuits included doing an occasional prerelease drug study for a pharmaceutical company. Another involved the opportunity to start to look at some of the systematic data that I had been collecting on independent psychiatric evaluations done for workers' compensation insurance carriers. I am convinced that many psychiatric diagnoses in this social setting have a different course compared with identical diagnoses in patients when financial secondary gain issues are not involved. By conducting a standardized psychiatric interview, along with rating scales and psychometric instruments, I have been able to collect data in a systematic fashion. Perhaps I will be able to make a small contribution to the development of the DSM-V or -VI.

To free up more time, I started scheduling regular patient office visits 3 out of 4 weeks each month. The fourth week was set aside to pursue research interests. Having 1 week per month dedicated solely to research and continuing education pursuits has not always been possible, and many times I have had to see emergency patients or consults during this week. It also gave me an opportunity to catch up on the paperwork generated by the psychiatric evaluations I was doing for third parties. This really took a lot of pressure off, and I do not at all miss the constant feeling of being behind.

Practice Hours

On Mondays and Wednesdays, I schedule office hours from 1:00 P.M. to 5:00 P.M. On Tuesdays and Thursdays, office hours are scheduled from 1:00 P.M. to 7:00 P.M. Frequently, patients will be added during the noon hour. I try to reserve Friday afternoons for depositions, urgent consultations, and catch-up.

In the office, during a typical week, I will see 30 patients for a short medication-check visit (10 to 15 minutes each), 3 patients for 25- to 30-minute visits for medication check and brief supportive psychotherapy, 2 patients for traditional 50-minute psychotherapy, 2 consultations for other physicians, and 9 patients who are in the process of workers' compensation psychiatric evaluations. In the hospital, I see an average of 3 patients.

The mornings are reserved for meetings, hospital rounds, and electroconvulsive therapy (ECT). ECT sessions are usually given Monday, Wednesday, and Friday. They start at 7:00 A.M. and are usually finished in an hour. Months will go by without any ECT; other times, we will treat three or four patients at a time. Hospital rounds usually start at 8:30 A.M. and end at about 11:30 A.M. When I was doing general psychiatry, this meant seeing the patient on the same day the referring physician believed was indicated, or if it was an emergency, within 48 hours. This availability quickly builds up a legion of referral sources, provides quick evaluation, and allows treatment to begin for the patients who need it. However, in very short order, it not only eats one's free time, but necessitates giving up other activities to make the time to see the patient. Quickly, one's hours become extended into the late evening and weekends. Although such a service is valuable, it becomes exhausting. Even if one gives up time for many other things and "squeezes" the extra patient in, one's vitality can soon be dissipated. One can easily become too tired to pursue other interests in psychiatry. Speed of response was helpful in establishing and building a large and successful practice. At this time, I believe my practice is maintained primarily through reputation for good work. I still attempt to help referral sources who need fast responses by referring to younger psychiatrists in the community who have time and are willing to provide fast response service.

Those who become "niche" psychiatrists and have expertise in a limited area can schedule patients at their convenience. Instead of seeing the patient within 48 hours, it would not be unusual to schedule the patient for an evaluation in 6 weeks. Of course, if there were other psychiatrists with similar expertise who would see the patient sooner, no one would wait the 6 weeks. Now, instead of working 70 to 80 hours a week doing routine psychiatry, I work 40 to 50 hours a week. For the most part, I am no longer mentally and physically exhausted after a day of work. I had built my practice and reputation for almost 20 years before switching to this type of practice. In retrospect, it probably would have been possible in my location after about 10 years if I had been more focused on subspecialty practice as a career goal.

In addition to the psychiatrist and psychologist making up the cost-sharing partnership with me, another full-time psychiatrist, two part-time psychiatrists, and four full-time psychiatric social workers work as independent practitioners in the office. One of the other psychiatrists is working on developing a niche in psychiatric managed care. The other professionals are generalists, although each has several areas of expertise. This group setting allows for interchange of ideas in addition to support and backup when necessary.

Office Overhead Cost Sharing

All of the general office expenses are divided three ways. The other professionals in the group pay a monthly fee for the use of office space and clerical support. The general office expenses include secretarial salaries, utilities, and supplies that are used by the entire office. Each professional is essentially in private practice but shares resources such as secretarial office support and equipment.

The office has clerical support staff from 8:30 A.M. to 5:30 P.M. Monday, Wednesday, and Friday and 8:30 A.M. to 7:30 P.M. on Tuesdays and Thursdays. Each professional sets his or her own hours and schedules his or her own patients. The patient fees are paid directly to the treating professional but collected by the secretarial staff if paid during regular office hours. Some patients may see two or more of the professionals in the office. Each professional has a separate chart for the patient. The accounting system keeps track of charges and payments separately.

The clinical psychologist oversees the general office management. Three full-time secretaries handle all of the clerical aspects of the office. Each secretary has a general area of responsibility, but each knows the others' job functions. One secretary concentrates on word processing, another on accounts receivable, and a third on scheduling. We also have a part-time receptionist who helps in answering the phone and greeting patients. Payment for professional services is expected and usually collected at each visit.

Because my individual practice is limited to evaluations and psychopharmacology, my routine differs significantly from the traditional mental health professional who sees one patient per hour.

Office Visits

First Visit

My first visit with a patient in the office is usually for one of three reasons:

1. A comprehensive psychiatric evaluation at the request of a nonmedical third party
2. A consultation for another medical or mental health professional
3. A patient referred from a nonmedical or mental health professional for treatment of a particular problem

A comprehensive psychiatric evaluation is usually done at the request of a nonmedical third party such as an insurance company or attorney to try to answer some specific questions and to possibly recommend a treatment program. A workers' compensation independent evaluation is a good example.

A workers' compensation evaluation would require three separate visits to my office. During the first visit, a psychiatric nurse would administer a series of standardized history-taking instruments and a select group of psychometric standardized tests. The patient typically spends 2 to 3 hours in the office completing these tests and is given several to take home and complete.

Second Visit

The second visit consists of a standard clinical psychiatric interview. I set aside 1½ hours for this visit. Between the second and third visit, I review and summarize all available medical records for the clinical record. I also score, interpret, and summarize the psychometric testing and standardized history instruments for the clinical record.

Third Visit

I set aside 1 hour for the third office visit. During this visit, I explore with the patient any additional information uncovered during the testing or review of medical records. If I make a psychiatric diagnosis, I formulate a treatment plan and discuss it with the patient. I dictate a summary letter answering the requested questions. The requesting party receives the summary letter plus an appendix and attachment. The appendix contains summaries of the two clinical visits and the review of medical records. The attachment contains the raw data from the psychometric testing and systematic history-taking instruments.

Traditional Consultation

I set aside 1 hour for a traditional consultation for a medical or mental health professional. The requesting professional receives a report containing a differential diagnosis and treatment alternatives. These treatment alternatives may include a recommendation about specific treatment strategies if the referring source is another psychiatrist. If the referring source is a family physician, I may suggest that the patient be referred to a psychiatrist or mental health professional. Also, if the referring physician is a family physician who is comfortable prescribing psychotropic medications, and it appears that this may be all that is necessary, a medical regimen may be outlined.

If the patient was referred for treatment, I outline a treatment plan as soon as I establish a diagnosis. This usually occurs after the first or second visit. If the patient has a psychiatric disorder that can be expected to respond to medication, the treatment plan usually requires short office visits for medication checks and telephone conferences in between the office visits. The interval between visits and telephone contacts depends on many factors, including type of medication and potential side effects.

Managed Care

During my residency training, emotionally unstable patients without psychosis were frequently seen in the emergency room in times of crisis. They were not admitted but referred to an outpatient treatment program. In my first few months of private practice, I followed the same approach with these patients. However, outpatient treatment was difficult to set up. The patients demanded a great deal of attention, time, and effort. Their insurance policies had very little, if any, coverage for outpatient benefits as compared with inpatient benefits. I soon realized that my colleagues were admitting these types of patients to an inpatient program. When I also began to do this, life became a lot easier for me. The inpatient program provided control and structure. The patients developed and strengthened support systems in a systematic fashion. The patients were able to start coping with the stresses they faced in everyday life.

At the time of discharge, the patient was off to a running start toward recovery. Outpatient treatment became much less demanding on me. Although the patient frequently had to pay a large part of the outpatient costs out of his or her own pocket, the outpatient service was much less intense and, hence, more affordable to the patient. In the residency training program, I treated indigent patients who did not have inpatient or outpatient insurance. However, many of the patients seen in private practice did have coverage for inpatient treatment but inadequate coverage for outpatient treatment. This type of treatment intervention worked well for the patient and myself, but at the cost of contributing to the escalation of hospital costs. As hospital costs rose, insurance premiums rose, and employers were finally pushed to looking for cheaper solutions. Hence, the birth of managed care.

Some managed programs have greatly increased the outpatient benefits so that patients can utilize a more intense outpatient treatment program. This ranges from seeing the patient on a daily basis for office visits to a partial hospitalization program in which the patient would spend the day at the hospital but sleep at home. Benefits such as these certainly allow more intensive treatment of the patient and still save on hospital costs.

Many managed care companies have not increased their benefits. However, they have developed strict criteria for inpatient admissions. Frequently, these criteria boil down to the patient being actively suicidal. From the moment the patient is no longer actively suicidal, these companies expect outpatient treatment to begin. This would often be a reasonable alternative to an inpatient program. However, without the insurance benefits to pay for such a program, most patients cannot afford to pay for it out of pocket. Government-supported clinics are not much help because, with their heavy patient load, patients cannot be seen on a daily basis. This becomes a real dilemma.

One cannot summarily say "the patient needs to stay in the hospital and get the proper treatment." If the insurance company disallows the patient's hospital stay, the patient becomes responsible for a huge bill. This can add tremendous pressures and stress that can further complicate a psychiatric disorder. In such situations, I find myself making compromises (i.e., explaining the alternatives to the patient and family). We then usually see the patient on the most intense basis possible utilizing nurse visits and telephone conferences. If there is enough support in the family, we have been successful. Thus far, I have not had any tragedies occur in such situations, but several patients have dropped out of treatment, and I do not have any data on how they are doing. As yet, I have found only minor deviation from "ideal" practice as a result of managed care. Furthermore, under economic pressure, I have found that certain alternatives to traditional treatment, such as shorter hospitalizations, may be just as efficacious. In any event, when the physician loses patience with the managed care process, it is the patients who suffer.

Financial survival in a managed care environment will require increased efficiency. Although allied mental health professionals functioning as counselors and psychotherapists is one route to cost-effective treatment, the utilization of a psychiatric nurse allows the psychiatrist to be more efficient by concentrating on what only he or she is qualified to do.

I have worked with psychiatric nurses, psychiatric nurse practitioners, master's degree psychiatric social workers, master's degree mental health counselors, and Ph.D. clinical psychologists. I prefer to work with psychiatric nurses. Such nurses who "moonlight" on a part-time basis in a psychiatrist's office may provide a transition for the psychiatrist to start working with this mental health professional. The advantage of employing nurses is their knowledge of medical illness and psychiatric disorders. They are more knowledgeable about psychotropic medication. This is particularly helpful in evaluating side effects. The psychiatric nurse practitioner, with more extensive training in medical and psychiatric assessment and psychopharmacology, can be even more helpful. Usually, the nurses have less psychotherapy/counseling training and experience than other mental health professionals. The weaknesses and strengths of the psychotherapist–counselors are often just the opposite of those of the psychiatric nurse. Familiarity with psychotropic and nonpsychotropic medication, including side effects and response times, enables them to effectively communicate with the patients and their families in these areas. Increased use of allied mental health professionals allows the psychiatrist to operate more efficiently.

Telephone Conferences

The telephone conference is an innovation that can be cost-effective and clinically important. It increases compliance, provides close monitoring for side effects, and allows more rapid drug titration. Costs are reduced by keeping actual office visits to a minimum. When starting the patient on a new medication or significant dose change, a telephone conference allows you to identify potential problems more quickly than waiting for the next visit. Years ago, before doing telephone conferences, the patients would frequently stop an antidepressant, and I would not learn about it until their next appointment. It takes long enough to get a response to an antidepressant without this delay. At the end of an office visit, I inform the patient that a telephone conference will take place at a given time and date. The patient's name is recorded in the nurse's appointment book for the day the call is scheduled to take place. The psychiatric nurse contacts the patient and completes the telephone conference form. I review the patient's responses. If I am unsure or unclear about some aspects of the report, I will contact the patient myself by telephone. Otherwise, I will write out instructions either to continue with the same medication or give specific instructions about changes in medication. In addition, the time for the next telephone conference may be established if the next office visit is not scheduled to occur in a timely fashion.

The telephone conference form (Table 10–1) serves several purposes.

Medication. The patient is asked to recite all the medication he or she is taking. Discrepancies are occasionally found between what the patient reports he or she is taking and what the office record indicates was prescribed. Reasons for discrepancies include the following:

• Misunderstanding of instructions
• A change in medication made by another physician
• The pills ran out and the patient did not want to get a refill until speaking with a psychiatrist at the next appointment
• A side effect occurred that "was not serious enough to bother you with"
• The pharmacy filled the wrong drug (e.g., doxidan instead of doxepin)

Care must be taken to explain the purpose of the double check to both the patient and the office staff responsible for performing the telephone conference. A new, overzealous, or overburdened nurse may complete the medication part of the form before calling the patient, to save time. The patient may then be asked to confirm what that chart indicates. This does not always work because the patient may erroneously agree to the nurse's recital. *Always* insist on the patient's reciting his or her medication.

Progress. Are target symptoms getting better or at least not getting worse? The sample telephone conference form contains some general target symptoms. Different forms containing target symptoms for specific diagnostic categories could be developed. (I initially called the telephone conference a progress report.)

Side effects. Occasionally, a patient is reluctant to report side effects. Frequently, a small adjustment will decrease the side effect or at least prevent it from worsening.

New problems. Give patients the opportunity to report new problem areas that may need to be resolved before the next scheduled appointment.

Table 10–1.   Telephone conference form

TELEPHONE CONFERENCE_____ DATE_____

PATIENT:_____ PHONE:_____

                                                        DRUGSTORE:_____

Medications: Name   Dose   Instructions

1)_____

2)_____

3)_____

4)_____

5)_____

6)_____

Date next APPT:_____   Enough meds next APPT: (Yes   No)

Changes since last contact: (Better   Worse   Same)

_____

_____

General spirits and mood: (Better   Worse   Same)

Appetite: (Better   Worse   Same)   (Increased   Decreased   Same)

Energy level: (Better   Worse   Same)

Sleep: (Better   Worse   Same)   (Initial   Interval   Terminal)

Any side effects: No   Yes_____

Any problems: No   Yes_____

Orders:

1)_____

2)_____

3)_____

4)_____

Patient called (   ) Changes charted (   ) Pharmacy called (   )
Charge posted (   )

                                        _____

                                                    By

Documentation. This demonstrates that the patient had been given opportunities to report adverse side effects or other problems in a systematic fashion.

Orders. A written record of order changes is noted in the office record. A time for an additional telephone conference may be noted in this section if one is indicated before the next scheduled visit.

At present, a psychiatric nurse is scheduled to be in the office to do telephone conferences on Monday and Friday morning from 9:00 A.M. to 12:00 P.M. and on Tuesday and Thursday evening from 4:30 P.M. to 7:00 P.M. The dates and times of the conferences are scheduled either during the last office visit or during the last phone conference. Patients also frequently call the office for an unscheduled phone conference during this time when they have some inquiries about nonemergent items. I will request that a progress report be completed whenever a patient misses an appointment so as to keep abreast of the patient's current state and to be able to reschedule the next appointment at an appropriate time.

Financial Issues

No patient has ever complained about the telephone conference itself. Some have complained about the charge for the service. I initially did not charge for the telephone conference. As my practice grew, it became an invaluable part of the patient management system. Unfortunately, my overhead was increasing considerably. In 1993, the additional surcharge for my malpractice insurance to have two nurses work part-time during the hours listed above was over $1,000 just for vicarious liability. The cost would have been the same for up to five full-time nurses. The nurses' malpractice insurance itself was only about $100.00 per nurse. Also, the expense of the nurses' salary and benefits has to be considered. I do not view the telephone conference as a method to make money, but I did want to "break even."

A charge was then instituted. At present, the charge for the routine telephone conference is $8.00. If we have many telephone conferences within a short time, I frequently will waive the charge. Charges are also waived on patients' requests because of financial problems.

Current Procedural Terminology (CPT) codes for the telephone conference are listed in Table 10–2.

Table 10–2. Current Procedural Terminology (CPT) codes for telephone calls

99371	Telephone call by a physician to a patient, or for consultation or medical management, or for coordinating medical management with other health care professionals; simple or brief, to clarify or alter previous instructions, to integrate new information from other health professionals into the medical treatment plan, or to adjust therapy.
99372	Intermediate, to provide advice to an established patient on a new problem, or to initiate therapy that can be handled on the phone, to discuss test results in detail, to coordinate medical management of a new problem in an established patient, to discuss and evaluate new information and details, or to initiate a new plan of care.
99373	Complex or lengthy counseling session with anxious or distraught patient, detailed discussion with family members regarding seriously ill patient, lengthy communication necessary to coordinate complex services of several different health care professionals working on different aspects of the total patient care plan.

Recent Medicare changes initially disallowed the telephone conference. However, by utilizing the telephone conference instead of an office visit, the charge is allowable, but not covered by Medicare. Patients are given a choice as to whether they want to come in for an office visit at more expense to the general health care system and more inconvenience to them personally, or have a telephone conference. Although it is not required that the patient sign a document of notification for a noncovered charge, it is our routine practice to do so because of the confusion generated in the Medicare reimbursement system. Table 10–3 contains one of the Health Care Financing Administration disclaimer forms a patient may sign in my office. Although the financial goal for the progress report was only to break even, I have not done so. The collections for the nurses' work will bring in about 60% of their cost, but they allow me to be available to more patients for diagnostic interviews, consultations, and/or treatment.

Table 10–3. Health Care Financing Administration disclaimer

Proof of notification required by the
Health Care Financing Administration

ADVANCE NOTICE FOR MEDICAL NECESSITY DENIALS

I have been notified that the following services are
not covered by Medicare.
I agree to be personally and fully responsible for payment.

1. Telephone conference/progress reports in lieu of a visit to the office.

2. Long-distance telephone charges.

3. Evening visit surcharges.

4. Missed visit charges.

5. Billing charges.

6. Interest charges.

7. Nonmedical visits (e.g., to talk about family member not in treatment, general background information).

8. Family medical psychotherapy without the patient being present.

9. Interpretation or explanation of results of psychiatric, or other medical examinations and procedures (other than for legal or consultative purposes) for other physicians, agencies, or insurance carriers.

10. Environmental intervention for medical management purposes on a psychiatric patient's behalf with agencies, employers, or institutions.

11. Preparation of report of patient's status, history, treatment, or progress (other than for legal or consultative purposes) for other physicians, agencies, or insurance carriers.

_____
Signature

_____
Date

Conclusion

It has been 20 years since my younger son was born with Down's syndrome. As he finishes his school training and is ready to receive more training in supported employment, I know that he was never the financial burden that I thought he would be and certainly is a joy and blessing in my life. My practice now allows the excitement and stimulation that comes from pursuing some limited research interests while having a busy private practice with the luxury of selecting patients. Who could ask for anything more?

Chapter 11

Practice of Consultation-Liaison Psychiatry

John D. Pro, M.D.
Vicki Burnett, R.N.

*I*n this chapter, we discuss issues that are relevant to building and maintaining a successful consultation-liaison service in a private practice setting. Information about diagnostic and technical aspects of the field abounds, as consultation-liaison psychiatry rapidly approaches formal subspecialty status within the American Board of Psychiatry and Neurology. We will not discuss these issues in this chapter, but rather, we will focus on practical aspects of the consultation process that make the psychiatrists' intervention successful and lead to the generation of further consults, to successful remuneration, and most of all, to the successful treatment of the patient's psychiatric problem.

The chapter is organized sequentially beginning with the first request for the consult and ending with the posthospital phase of the consultation. We have also tried to address financial issues in consultation psychiatry, and we have stressed the importance of the psychiatrist as the leader of the mental health team.

What Is a Successful Consultation?

Many believe that a psychiatric consult should be performed in the consultant's spare time and is essentially a service those who are in private practice must perform. These people believe that success is achieved by minimizing the time and effort of consults so that more time is available for a more lucrative and more interesting practice. Others see a consultation as successful only if it leads to 100% reimbursement in a fee-for-service system. These people are disappointed when consultations do not always generate this percentage of payment. On the other hand, psychiatrists, such as ourselves, deem a consultation successful when, not only do the patient and the family feel better, but also when the consult generates other business for the psychiatrist's general practice, including the office practice and psychiatric hospital practice. If consultations become a large part of one's private practice in general, and if a substantial number of office patients can be generated through consultation, the psychiatrist will have vested interest in maintaining high quality. We have oriented the chapter to this group of practitioners.

Maintaining a Successful Consultation Practice

A successful office practice is necessary to maintain a successful consultation practice. Many patients seen in the hospital may benefit from longer-term follow-up in the office. Many of these patients may benefit from psychotherapy and/or medications. Others also may benefit from brief inpatient stays in a psychiatric unit or a private psychiatric hospital. Integrating consultation-liaison work with general psychiatric practice, then, is really the ultimate goal. A psychiatrist probably cannot work exclusively in consultation-liaison psychiatry and be successful in private practice.

Obviously, one must be dedicated and interested in the field of consultation-liaison psychiatry to be successful. I became interested in consultation-liaison work while doing my residency in general psychiatry. There, I had the opportunity to learn from many excellent teachers, all of whom believed that psychiatry is a part of medicine. Because of my interest in the field, I was fortunate to be in one of the first classes of National Institute of Mental Health Consultation-Liaison Fellows.

After the fellowship, I went on to complete a residency in neurology. Both of these postgraduate experiences prepared me well for my current work in medical psychiatry. I will never regret the extra training, but I believe that any well-trained general psychiatrist with a thoughtful, communicative, practical approach to the patient can perform an excellent consultation. The excitement of working with colleagues of all specialties and the rewards of helping physically sick people with emotional complications make the work meaningful to me.

My particular private practice consists of approximately 50% geriatric patients and 50% nongeriatric adult patients. Much of the consultation work increasingly is in the geriatric age range. I tend to see consults early in the morning to maximize my exposure to other doctors and to generate business. Many psychiatrists may find themselves avoiding the hospital at this time for various reasons, but I think it is important to maintain this visibility in order to generate further consultations and to maximize face-to-face communication with doctors. It is much easier to coordinate the care at this time of day because everyone is available on the wards. During the second half of the morning, I make rounds at a private psychiatric hospital located on the campus of the general hospital. In the afternoon, I see office patients, but I make every effort to return to the general hospital to see any emergency consults at least briefly. I see a large number of new patients each week, and my practice tends to be a fifty-fifty blend of psychotherapy and medication patients.

However, in private practice, the distinction between "therapy" patients and "medication" patients is blurred and tends to be artificial. I render some type and degree of therapy to every patient I see. Furthermore, I rarely see a "medication" patient for less than 20 to 30 minutes. Treating the family of the patient has been an increasing part of my practice as managed care and other pressures mount to "cure" the patient more quickly. These principles apply both in consultation work and in the psychiatric hospital.

Three General Principles

The first general principle is that a psychiatrist cannot have a successful consultation practice unless he or she views himself or herself as part of a medical team and takes an active interest in the medical problems of the patient. Psychiatrists' unique perspective results from having an interest in the patient's medical or surgical problem as well as their psychiatric problem; this enables the psychiatrist to make a significant difference in the patient's care.

Second, note that in every phase of the consultation process, the greatest determinant of success is effective communication. Ongoing communication with nurses, social workers, clergy, and the patient and family as well as the attending physician cannot be overemphasized. Effective communication helps to destigmatize psychiatric interventions, minimize countertransference, build trust and confidence in the psychiatrist as the expert in mental health care, make the psychiatrist's intervention much more effective, and allow the psychiatrist to be more efficient.

A final principle is related to diagnostic issues. Although diagnosis in consultation psychiatry is not the topic of this chapter and can be found elsewhere in the large body of literature in the field, two points are relevant to a successful consultation practice. First, DSM-IV (American Psychiatric Association 1994) criteria for psychiatric illness should be part of the consultation psychiatrist's repertoire and are very important in assessing patients. Nonetheless, when communicating with other staff and medical personnel, DSM-IV criteria are often too cumbersome and too incongruous with medical terminology to be used rigidly. If these criteria and other complex psychological terminology are used, then the meaning should be explained to the physician. The simpler and more practical the terminology, the more effective the consultation will become. Second, to be successful, the consultation psychiatrist must be familiar with a wide variety of medical illnesses and their impact on the psyche. By far, the most important of these is the syndrome of delirium. This problem is so common and so frequently misdiagnosed by nonpsychiatrists that a psychiatrist really cannot be successful in his or her practice without being able to recognize, evaluate, and treat the delirious patient.

In summary, successful consultation practice requires a number of key ingredients. Certainly, the physician's attitude that he or she is part of the medical team and the conviction that the consultation can make a difference in the patient's care are critical. Communication with all those involved in the consultation including the patient, the family, and the staff is critical. The consultation psychiatrist must have a very sophisticated medical and psychiatric diagnostic repertoire, must be able to communicate in simple, practical language, and must be an expert in the diagnosis and treatment of delirium.

Receiving the Consultation

Success in consultation begins with a proper reception of the consult. The staff answering the phone should be trained in what to say and what type of information to obtain when a consultation is delivered to the office. For example, the receptionist should politely ask the person delivering the message if the patient needs to be seen right away or if the referring physician would like to speak with the psychiatrist about the consultation. If the physician calls with the consult, then the psychiatrist should talk personally with the doctor because, if it is important enough for the doctor to call, the psychiatrist should consider it his or her obligation to respond directly. A physician who calls a psychiatrist's office and communicates a consult to an uninterested or hurried receptionist is unlikely to call again.

The receptionist, at some point, should also attempt to obtain the patient's insurance information, either from the referring staff or by calling the ward secretary in the hospital. Most health personnel are accustomed to discussing insurance issues and do not mind such questions. One exception might be requests to nurses in the intensive care unit who are themselves quite hurried and who expect rapid responses from other consultants with "no questions asked." Information about insurance can prevent awkward consultations for patients who are members of health maintenance organizations or whose insurance companies have a panel of psychiatrists who are expected to answer requests for consults.

After receiving the consultation, if there is any question about the patient or the need for emergency care, it would be diplomatic for the psychiatrist to call the floor directly and ask the nurses if there are any particular problems that must be addressed immediately. At that time, the psychiatrist can also inform the nurses when to expect the consultation.

In summary, having a courteous office staff taking the initial consultation information and trying to communicate back to the floor prior to the consultation are both important steps toward a successful consultation.

Performing the Consultation

Seeing the patient within the first 24 hours of the consultation request, and preferably sooner, is an important ingredient of success in consultation. Furthermore, trying to see consultation patients in the morning when other physicians are making their rounds can be extremely helpful in communicating the psychiatrist's impressions of the patients, establishing the psychiatrist as part of the health care team, ensuring the psychiatrist's visibility, and communicating that the psychiatrist believes the consultations are important enough to take priority in their schedule.

After reviewing the chart, it is advisable to talk with the staff before seeing the patient. Family and medical issues can all be elucidated by discussing the patient with the nurses before performing the consultation. The nurses' perspective allows the psychiatrist to sense the patient's problem and gain some insight into the degree of resistance and stigma the patient may have in order to determine how much time he or she will have to spend overcoming these problems. If one can be effective in this area, the chances of payment are greater. Patients who feel they did not receive any help or who remain defensive toward psychiatric intervention throughout the hospitalization are less likely to pay their bill. Many patients, in fact, are not aware that the psychiatrist has been consulted at all. It helps, therefore, to know this information before entering the room. This is especially important with heart patients and patients in the intensive care unit who may fear being told that something is "all in their head" or that they are weak and unable to cope. In fact, it is probably best for the psychiatrist to assume that patients will be defensive and apprehensive and start from that point.

Defensiveness can be alleviated further by saying something like, "I often work with Dr. Joe, and I see a lot of his patients." The psychiatrist can ask the patient whether the doctor notified him or her about the consultation request and what his or her understanding is of the reason for the consult. Soon after entering the room, the consultant should always try to sit down in a chair or at the bedside.

It is always best to begin by asking the patient to talk about his or her experiences during the hospitalization and by taking a history of present medical illness. If the family is present, they usually should be invited to participate in the interview. After focusing on the medical illness, the psychiatrist can move more gracefully into the psychological arena. An attitude of empathy and concern for the person's physical suffering and an emphasis on symptom relief should always prevail during the consultation.

At the end of the consultation, it is important to ask patients what they think they need and how they think the psychiatrist might be able to help them. They should be invited to express their concerns about the stigma of seeing a psychiatrist, the stigma of not being able to manage things by themselves, and the stigma of the need for medications. I usually leave my business card with the patient and always reassure him or her that I will return, that I will share our discussion with his or her physician, and that I will speak with his or her family (unless they request differently). This helps to maximize the effectiveness of the consultation and also to minimize the tendency of many patients when they receive their bill to say, "I never asked for the psychiatrist." I usually discuss insurance issues briefly at the end of the consultation or at the end of the second visit. I emphasize that I intend to make the intervention "something that he or she can afford." Patients commonly ask the consultant whether he or she participates in Medicare. I always reassure the patient that I am "a Medicare doctor" and that I am not interested in "running up a big bill." I will return to the insurance issue later in this chapter. Finally, it is advisable to terminate the consultation at any point if the patient expresses that he or she does not want a psychiatrist.

In summary, to be effective, the consultant must assess the degree of resistance and stigma inherent in the consultation. This can be done by discussing the case beforehand with the nurses and by presenting oneself in as nonthreatening a fashion as possible with the patient and his or her family. Successful consultation depends on communicating the results with the nursing staff and eliciting their help in managing the patient's problems, especially with difficult patients. It is also important to communicate carefully and directly to the referring physician and to ensure that the physician approves of the type of intervention and that the consultant understands the physician's expectations of the consultation.

Communicating the Results

It is always important to speak with the staff following a consultation. This "mini inservice" serves a number of purposes. First, it is a liaison activity and builds rapport with the nursing staff. These discussions also allow for countertransference issues to be addressed, demystify what the psychiatrist is trying to do, and allow the psychiatrist to solicit the nurses' help in treating the patient's psychological problem. Many nurses ask "What can we say to the patient?"; having an inservice provides an opportunity for the consultant to help them understand the most effective interventions.

After the consultation, it is usually advisable to call the referring physician and briefly discuss the consultant's impressions and treatment plan. Again, it is best to use the most practical and simple language possible. Many referring physicians may be sensitive to or threatened by psychiatric intervention; calling the physician at this point allows the consultant to clarify how involved the referring doctor wants the psychiatrist to be. It may be necessary to ask the referring physician what he or she expected regarding the consultation. Most physicians will be open about this. Some referring physicians simply want the psychiatrist to prescribe antidepressants or to rule out any severe psychopathology. Others would like the consultant to completely take over the psychological care of the patient. This type of communication is particularly important in the areas of neurology, rehabilitation, family practice, general medicine, and, increasingly, on pain services where clinical activities and expertise often overlap.

After talking with the physician, the consultant should dictate a complete report, again trying to minimize the use of unnecessary jargon. If DSM-IV criteria are used, an explanation should follow. The consultant's impression and diagnosis should be summarized in the chart, and he or she should thank the referring physician for the consultation.

In the report and the chart, the consultant's plans for treatment should be listed carefully. This list should be comprehensive and should include, for example, the recommendation for hearing aids, laboratory tests, medications, talking with the family, and a social service consultation. All of these modes should be carried out, and the psychiatrist should try to follow up and report results in the ensuing progress notes. This will establish the psychiatrist as not only the coordinator of the psychiatric care, but also as an advocate for comprehensive care. It is always advisable for consultants who write orders in the chart to obtain the referring physician's approval.

Follow-up

The patient should be followed in the hospital as often as the consultant believes that it is necessary. Progress notes should be written clearly and should address the psychiatrist's comprehensive treatment plan. Again, in follow-up it is important to ask the nurses how the patient is doing and to try including them in the overall psychological management of the patient's symptoms. Including clergy and social workers is also desirable. It is also important to call the family to update them on the progress of a patient, especially when the patient is dying, is in a great deal of pain, or has other kinds of significant distress. By keeping in touch with the family, the consultant obtains their impressions of the patient's progress and explains how the family can be maximally helpful to the patient.

Assessing the timing of the follow-up visits is also important. The patient should not be seen unnecessarily, yet frequently enough for the consultant to be effective. The psychiatrist must not appear "money hungry." When I am unsure, I call the physician to ask him or her to recommend how often it would be helpful for me to stop by. Likewise, I always call the physician when I have completed the case; I explain my final recommendations and emphasize psychiatric follow-up.

Aftercare

The patient's psychiatric problem often requires longer-term care and more elaborate disposition planning than the medical problem. Aftercare can be complicated by many factors, including indigent patients, poor family support, and living out of town. As the head of the treatment team, the psychiatrist must be able to utilize a wide variety of resources to help these different patients and should not be afraid to treat indigent patients. The psychiatrist should prepare some type of disposition for each patient even if this means simply a request for a follow-up call "prn" for any further psychiatric problems. This follow-up should be carefully communicated to the staff and to the attending physician. Many patients seen in consultation may be suitable for follow-up in the psychiatrist's office and, in fact, many referring doctors may prefer this because they can follow the patient's psychological progress more closely. It is always advisable to tell the patients as they are about to leave the hospital, or if the consultant is "signing off," that they may call the consultant at any time if they have problems or questions.

If the consultation and the care have been complicated in any way, it is advisable to write letters to the referring physicians. This builds referrals and provides better continuity of care. If the patients are seen in the consultant's office, follow-up letters should be written periodically. With physicians who may be sensitive to psychiatrists "stealing the patient," it is even more important to clarify the psychiatrist's goals and reassure the referring doctor that they will remain in charge of the patient's care.

Reimbursement Issues

A common stereotype in consultation practice is that reimbursement for the work is poor. Actually, if the consultant is successful in maintaining a large number of consults, the number of paying consults will significantly outweigh those who do not pay. It is important for the consultant to discuss insurance reimbursement for psychiatric coverage with the patient at some point during the consultation. Consultants must be prepared to see indigent patients, however. In our practice, 20%–30% of the patients may be indigent or on Medicaid. Usually, consultations are covered under the major medical plans and are outside of the inpatient psychiatric benefits that tend to be more restrictive because of managed care. Preauthorization may be necessary for some consultations, when required by managed care companies; this authorization should be obtained as early as possible.

It is probably desirable for consultation psychiatrists to participate in Medicare and Medicaid as well as other common managed care plans such as Blue Cross because they will encounter a wide variety of patients with different insurance coverage in the general hospital setting. Medicare does require an authorization signature from the patient, and I use signature cards routinely, shortly after the first consultation. I simply tell the patient that his or her signature is required by Medicare so that I can file the Medicare claim, and I reassure the patient that my office will take care of all of the paperwork. This usually is reassuring, rather than upsetting, to the patient.

In terms of Medicaid, it is important to ask the patient if his or her Medicaid is current and, if not, to have social services help reinstate the assistance. Many indigent patients are eligible for Medicaid after they have been in the hospital for several weeks. Helping patients to obtain these benefits can at least provide some reimbursement for the consult. In other patients who, at first glance, do not appear to have insurance, a call to the hospital business office or a direct question to the patient may reveal that they have reasonable private insurance. In all cases, an aggressive approach aimed at understanding the patient's coverage is essential and can reduce write-offs.

Large general hospitals increasingly employ managed care nurses, and they can help the consultant obtain authorization and coverage on policies that might superficially deny reimbursement to a consulting psychiatrist. The referring doctor's office will often be able to send necessary referral forms authorizing consultation and follow-up in the general hospital even though the psychiatrist is "out of work" with the particular insurance plan. Most managed care companies will pay the consultant for services in the general hospital in my experience. Holding the patient responsible for the difference between the insurance allowable and the psychiatrist's fee is a matter of judgment and discretion and should be approached on a case-by-case basis.

Reimbursement issues, especially in an atmosphere of managed care, can be frustrating. However, knowing the patient's insurance plan and helping him or her to obtain Medicaid coverage, if indicated, can alleviate some of these frustrations.

Utilizing hospital resources and the referring physician's business office can also enhance reimbursement. This aggressive stance toward insurance issues can often raise reimbursement to the same level as that in the psychiatric hospital and in the private office. In fact, with the exception of the indigent patients, the reimbursement for general hospital patients is approximately the same as it is for patients in the private psychiatric hospital. The codes and the reimbursement rates are the same. When patients who have been seen in any hospital setting and with whom one has rapport come to the office, they may be more motivated to pay their portions of the hospital bill and the office call.

It is also important to keep in mind that in consultation work, the use of time codes for psychotherapy or family therapy legitimately include the time spent coordinating the treatment of the patient with nurses, visiting nurses, and social workers. This extra time can, indeed, be billed as psychotherapy. In addition, using these resources allows the consultation psychiatrist to be more efficient and to see more consults than would be possible without these personnel. Indirectly, the volume of consults that an efficient consultant can generate often compensates for the write-off. At our hospital, we are fortunate to have a psychiatric care team composed of two psychiatric nurses, one of whom assisted in organizing this chapter. These psychiatric nurses are increasingly common in large general hospitals and are extremely valuable, not only in terms of patient care, but also in terms of raising the level of awareness of mental health issues in the hospital personnel.

As a result of the efforts of these nurses, the general staff nurses have become much more sophisticated psychologically. We also utilize visiting nurses to provide continuity of psychiatric care in the patient's home after he or she is discharged. All of these resources help the psychiatrist provide the best care possible for the patient at the lowest cost and with the highest efficiency.

Liaison Activities

Liaison activities should be a part of any successful consultation practice. Liaison activities help build referrals and help establish the psychiatrist as the leader of the mental health team and as an expert in psychological treatment. Common liaison activities include pain clinics, cardiovascular services, and renal and transplant services. Increasingly, ethics committees provide an important forum for the liaison psychiatrist as well. Talks to the medical staff at noon conferences and inservices for nurses, especially about direct patient care issues, can lead to more referrals and ultimately make the psychiatrist's job easier by diffusing the care.

At every juncture of the consultation process, there is an opportunity to ensure the success of the consultation. We have outlined the important areas in this chapter. The attitude of the psychiatrist, the ability to communicate with other professionals, and the use of available resources are essential features of successful consultation in a private practice setting.

Reference

American Psychiatric Association: Diagnostic and Statistical Manual of Mental Disorders, 4th Edition. Washington, DC, American Psychiatric Association, 1994

Chapter 12

Practice of Addiction Psychiatry

Neil Goldman, M.D.

*D*uring my residency training in psychiatry, addiction psychiatry was not foremost on my list of future careers. My initial training and exposure to addicted patients was not a rewarding experience, reflecting the negative attitudes and beliefs of my supervisors toward addictive disorders. As a result, I did not specifically consider addiction psychiatry as a future career choice. Fortunately, my early negative introduction to the addictions field was balanced both by the positive personal experience I had working with these patients and also by later positive reinforcement by leaders in the field with whom I had the pleasure of working. My 2-year obligation to the military exposed me to clinical experiences that proved instrumental in establishing my future career. Fortunately, my assignment was at Pease Air Force Base, where I became the chief of a small outpatient mental health clinic. This experience helped contribute to my career choice in many ways. Our staffing mimicked a traditional outpatient psychiatric program. In addition to myself, there was a psychologist, a social worker, two psychiatric technicians, and a clinic secretary. Our patient population was drawn from both active and retired military personnel and their families. The opportunity to design and implement treatment programs and to practice varying styles of clinical psychiatry was ever-present. I was able to experience, in a quasi-private setting, individual, family, and group approaches. We conducted educational groups and experimented with group intakes to expedite entrance into our treatment programs. In all, I had the opportunity to compare private-style treatment approaches with clinic services that could be administered to large groups of patients.

In this setting, I was exposed to many patients with alcohol- and drug-related problems and, by necessity, mastered the diagnosis and treatment of these disorders. I began to identify how they influenced and caused a wide range of psychiatric disorders. In fact, in most clinical situations to which I was exposed, substance-related problems and their complications were very common. I was fascinated with the denial (at that time I saw it as deceit) of the patients and the elaborate extent to which they would go to protect their drinking. I began to increasingly focus on these problems and gradually realized that I was, in fact, "subspecializing."

Alcoholism and Addictions Psychiatry

Often, residents are not well prepared in the area of alcoholism and addictions. Residents bring many interfering biases and stereotypes into their training. Often, psychiatry itself is seen as being on the fringe of medicine. Addiction psychiatry may then be the fringe on the fringe. Colleagues who practice outside this area of specialization often ask if I enjoy working with "drunks." Despite their intellectual awareness, they most often forget that alcoholic patients and even most drug-addicted people start out with an intact social support system and are productive members of society. Only if we delay intervention until the late stages of their illness does the classical, although archaic, image of the "down-and-out" alcoholic person present itself. We may even say that it is through the primary physician's inability to adequately interface with the patient and his or her addiction that the problem intensifies.

The alcoholism and addictions field has a wide range of treatment settings to offer prospective patients. They range from hospital-based detoxifications to social setting sobering-up stations. They may include various rehabilitation programs and halfway houses. Much work is also done in outpatient settings that have a wide range of services and therapeutic modalities, including individual and group counseling, supportive psychotherapy, family therapy, and vocational services.

How does the individual psychiatrist fit into this schema? First, some patients prefer a private setting to a clinic setting or a private psychiatrist to an individual with lesser credentials. Many patients are apprehensive about groups, including Alcoholics Anonymous, and seek out a more individualized approach to their problems. Another potential advantage of the psychiatrist is that he or she is in a unique position to interface with other medical specialists and to assess atypical presentations of the disease. Comorbid psychiatric disorders with alcoholism or other addictions fit especially well into the psychiatrist's clinical domain.

With a developing concept of what type of practice I envisioned for myself (i.e., private clinical practice combined with an academic appointment), I was able to determine what I needed after my discharge from the military. My desire for a lifestyle that included marriage, children, and a strong commitment to family life led to my decision to relocate back to the New York City area, which was my original home. With these factors in mind, I was able to locate a postpsychiatric residency fellowship in alcoholism.

Fellowships in Addiction Psychiatry

Pursuing fellowship training offered many advantages for me. Of primary importance was the actual specialized training and the opportunity to meet other professionals and experts in the field. Through this exposure, I could more easily keep abreast of trends in the addiction field and establish myself within this subspecialty. I also had to consider the downside of doing a fellowship. It is, after all, an additional year (sometimes 2 years) of not beginning a private practice or a full-time salaried position. In my particular situation, I was willing to extend my training, not only for the reasons outlined above, but also to allow time for relocation. After all, I was moving back to New York City after 2 years away, and the fellowship year was very important in establishing connections and allowing for a more deliberate decision regarding my future career plans.

Fellowships in addiction psychiatry were very rare when I was entering the field; now, there are many more, and they range from the traditional fifth postgraduate year of training, with a mix of clinical, administrative, and educational involvements, to those that are essentially junior attending positions. My choice of a fellowship enabled me to subspecialize and to reestablish myself in an academic setting in the community of my choice. At the same time, I was able to begin a private practice, compare that experience with the one in the military, and begin to identify the specifics of practice that interested me.

Development of a Private Clinical Practice

I further clarified my goals toward developing a private clinical practice, with a focus on self-paying private patients, in the addictions field. This was balanced by an active involvement with a hospital-based clinic patient population. I did not want to sacrifice the academic and teaching opportunities offered in a training hospital, which I felt were an integral part of a well-rounded career. I worked full-time in a teaching hospital running an addiction consultation service to the general hospital. Salaried positions in addiction psychiatry are becoming more readily available as the field in general is moving into the mainstream of psychiatry. This position further solidified my position within the subspecialty and brought me in contact with large numbers of professional staff and physicians in the hospital. I began to be seen as a psychiatrist with subspecialty interests in the addictions. Even working full-time, it was possible for me to begin to nurture my private practice.

Just as the choice of affiliation with a well-established and acclaimed hospital is important in determining professional contacts and opportunities, a private office must be well located and appointed to attract privately paying patients. I had to decide whether to establish a "Park Avenue" address or one that afforded an image of respectability and status through association with an institution. I chose to solidify my affiliation with the hospital in an attempt to draw on professional resources that would naturally be present in such a setting. Being relatively new, it was important to establish my presence as early as possible by being available, flexible, and capable of serving the needs of the physicians in my institution. This meant being available for consults at any time, weekdays and weekends, both in and out of the hospital. Even though my primary interest was to see patients with alcoholism or addictions, I was called to see a full range of psychiatric problems. I accepted this opportunity to provide a broad range of services to the referring physicians, but also used it to inform them of my primary interest and focus. Providing these consults also meant seeing some of the most difficult patients to work with, either because of the specific diagnosis, personality disorder, inability to pay, or previous rejection by other more experienced psychiatrists.

What I find most important in maintaining a satisfied core of referring physicians is to provide good clinical care to their patients.

The best referral source is a patient reporting back to his or her physician that he or she is satisfied and benefiting from the treatment. Keep in mind that it is not possible for the psychiatrist, especially one with an office-based psychodynamically oriented practice, to reciprocate numerically. The service we offer that is most important to the internist or surgical specialist is that we can help them in an area of medicine in which their knowledge, skills, or interests may be limited. It is more important to present to them as a knowledgeable, competent, and accommodating specialist than to seek a quid pro quo in numbers.

During these early formative years, it was important that I remain busy yet available and accommodating yet ever more discriminating to allow me to move in the direction that I established as a goal for my clinical practice. At times, it was enticing to be more flexible and flow with the availability of private practice opportunities as opposed to remaining somewhat selective in terms of my chosen subspecialty. Sometimes, these opportunities proved illusory.

At one point early in establishing my practice, I was enticed by the availability of a large number of Medicare referrals from a nursing home. It seemed that all of a sudden many patients required psychiatric consultation and treatment. I began to question whether my choice of subspecialization, addiction psychiatry, should be replaced by geriatrics. There was an abundance of referrals and clinical work; a Medicare-based practice was not what I had envisioned, but it might be financially rewarding. For months I consulted and treated patients in the nursing home. I generated and submitted Medicare forms for reimbursement. After approximately 4 months, the consults stopped, and I was confused. I knew it was not related to the quality of my clinical work. At about that time, the Medicare reimbursement forms started coming in, and the situation immediately became clear. Most of the claims paid little or nothing because of the patient's yearly deductible. I later learned that the physicians who provided the bulk of the ongoing care to the nursing home patients delayed submitting their claims until the "consultants" exhausted the patient's deductible.

This was not just a case of being deceived by my fellow physicians, but rather an opportunity to reexamine my own interests, needs, and goals. It became clear to me how important it is to stay focused on one's own priorities even when other enticing opportunities come along. The most important opportunities have always been those that allowed me to develop a professional identity and expertise. Repeated focus on educating the referring physicians as to how I could be of help to them proved most important in developing my subspecialized career. By providing early liaison efforts and educating our referral network that early intervention succeeds, we are best able to help our colleagues, their patients, and those who are referred to us for specialized treatment. As my practice grew, the growth itself forced additional change. As time is limited, building up an office-based private practice meant limiting other clinical involvements. I chose to stay with my salaried academic position and keep a limited, but selective, private practice. The challenge was to maintain a solid referral base while restricting some of my availability. An increase in my office-based private practice meant less time for consults or hospital-based care, which, in turn, meant less flexibility and availability to referring physicians.

Treatment Aspects

As my private office practice increased, I focused more on the important treatment aspects of an alcoholism and addiction psychiatry subspecialization. We do not work with patients in a vacuum. Unless we restrict treatment to patients with end-stage illness, we are invariably coordinating our treatment efforts in a systems approach. Treatment will focus on the patient but in combination with the family, significant others, employer, and/or private physician. Even though the type of therapy will be primarily individual in the private office setting, coordinating therapeutic efforts with all of the significant people in the patient's life not only represents good clinical care but also assures a steady referral network.

The growth of my private practice was not passive. As my practice approached 20 hours per week in time commitments, it became easier to select those patients I was willing to see in my practice. This meant working long hours, as I still maintained my full-time salaried position. Although it might be very difficult to maintain a full-time office-based addiction practice, it should be possible to build up to about 20 hours weekly within 4 to 5 years in my geographic area. I focused mostly on patients who had an intact family or social system to work with. This could be immediate or extended family, concerned friends or significant others, or even employers. I performed some consultations in my office and focused mostly on those individuals who were likely to warrant and follow through with active treatment.

Establishing practice goals is easy in comparison to adhering to them. For example, when screening calls from potential referral sources, it is important to be able to say "no," or at least to qualify what you can and are willing to provide in terms of professional service. Being everything to everybody may please nobody and, in fact, actually interfere with the growth of your practice. The most obvious compromise is one of volume of practice. There may be a need to turn down referrals that do not contribute to the growth of your ideal practice, but by doing so you will be better able to educate your referral sources as to the specifics of your practice style. Saying "yes" to a referral that does not advance your practice will only send an ambiguous message and slow your ability to develop your desired practice. In time though, the quantity of referrals will increase, and the initial trade-off in volume will be corrected.

Professional contact can and should be maintained in a wide variety of ways. Keep in mind that a seemingly successful practice that leads to increasing professional isolation may soon run out of steam. Developing professional contacts through academic, political, or professional organizations is very important. Often, several may be combined without excessive time being taken away from direct patient care. Local American Psychiatric Association committees and activities help the private practitioner maintain contact with others in the field. Establishing cross-specialty ties, specifically with medical specialists, helps diversify your potential referral base. Subspecialty conferences are an excellent way to keep abreast of developments in the field, but may not offer much in the way of referrals.

At first, I experimented with different treatment approaches. I tried a psychodynamic model, a family treatment model, and even a counseling model in conjunction with a 12-step approach. I learned that an eclectic approach, utilizing many aspects of the above models, was necessary. Patients with addictive disorders may require a very directive approach in the beginning, often involving their family as a supportive network. As they progress in treatment, other personality and neurotic issues surface, and a psychodynamic approach may be necessary.

About one-third of my patients have a comorbid Axis I disorder, usually depression, or a comorbid personality disorder. As most of my patients are fairly functional, personality disorders are generally of the less severe types, with few cluster A or borderline disorders. In the remaining two-thirds, the major tasks are to help the patient get the addiction under control first, and then to help them address the interpersonal problems and problems in living that arose because of the addiction. Thus, much of the psychotherapeutic work involves helping the patient to change maladaptive addiction-related behaviors and adjust to living a life free of substance abuse.

Relationships With Other Mental Health Professionals

An aspect of treatment that is more complicated than dealing with referring physicians is the complex relationships with other mental health professionals. Referrals from other psychiatrists are usually straightforward. They either want relief through transferring the patient for treatment, or they are seeking a second opinion and referral back. Other mental health workers may not be so explicit in their requests. There may be hidden agendas and/or fears that a patient referred for evaluation and psychopharmacotherapy may be enticed to switch therapists. This is especially so with patients in which the degree of clinical difficulty requires fairly close monitoring by the psychiatrist. In turn, this raises the question of which therapist is most capable of providing the comprehensive treatment required, thereby creating a conflict between the referring therapist and the consultant. Referrals to psychiatrists may also be designed to get a formal diagnosis so that the referring therapist may be eligible for insurance reimbursement. There is nothing wrong in this scenario if the parties involved are both aware of the true nature of the referral and the extent of the expected involvement for each. Another complicating aspect of the referral process is that the mental health professional may need to defuse the intensity of treatment in potentially litigious situations and protect themselves with a "deep pocket" physician as a cotherapist.

All these potential problem areas are real but do not negate the straightforward requests for cotreatment or consultation. The collaborative agreements that worked best for me were those that allowed for clarity in the working relationship. I tried to inform those I collaborated with as to the type and intensity of my practice style and whether I thought I could be of help to the referring mental health professional. I learned to steer clear of referrals from those who were not interested in understanding my practice style. The best collaboration for me was a loosely structured one that allowed for a case-by-case decision regarding my acceptance of the patient for consultation or treatment. Those referring specialists who accepted what I had to offer soon referred selectively and more appropriately.

Is collaboration good and competition bad for a private practice? It is not clear or simple. Some collaboration, especially if it locks you into a practice style that conflicts with your goals, may interfere with your progress toward the ideal. For example, if you are trying to establish a practice with a family treatment approach, accepting referrals for consultations only or individual patients without a support system will only increase your commitments in undesirable areas of practice and not further the growth of your idealized practice. On the other hand, competition may enable you to identify your primary interest and focus in therapy, thereby actually assisting the growth of an office-based practice. Educating your peers about your specific areas of interest (e.g., a family treatment approach) can actually change what appears to be a competitive climate into a collaborative one, especially when your peer is actively seeking more individual patients or consultation requests.

Managed Care

Once your practice is established, third-party oversight may play an increasing role. How to handle third-party payers begins with the issue of whether you would rather interface with the insurance carriers directly or with the patients themselves. How accommodating you are in accepting third-party payment determines the amount of interference. Clearly establishing an office policy of expecting payment directly from the patient with insurance reimbursement going to them will simplify and clarify responsibilities for payment. Complicating factors may involve patients who cannot afford the established fee, but clarifying the payment expectations may lead to discussions and subsequent fee reductions when appropriate. Maintaining separate financial arrangements (i.e., physician-patient and patient-insurance company rather than a triangulated arrangement of physician-patient-insurance company) will help keep the fee payment as a therapeutic issue. It is difficult to maintain a practice of only self-paying patients, especially if you are in a full-time private practice. Because my time was divided between a salaried position and a private practice, my full income was not dependent on either practice alone, and I had fewer hours to be filled; thus, I had more flexibility in choosing patients. As such, I have had greater success in maintaining a self-pay private practice. The proportion of self-pay private patients increased steadily for me over time. At least half of my private patients at any time are at full fee and make their payments directly. The other half may be at a somewhat reduced rate or may utilize insurance reimbursements to cover some of the bill.

Managed care clearly has influenced my practice. Some patients do not make an appointment because their insurance policy requires them to go through a "gatekeeper." Some patients must have prior approval with a preapproved psychiatrist, and others discover that they will not be reimbursed except under very limited conditions. However, many patients with little or no insurance coverage are willing to meet the financial expense on their own. Some patients are unwilling to utilize their insurance coverage for privacy reasons and are also willing to pay out of pocket. It is also possible, especially with patients who are competent employees, to arrange for the employer to assume responsibility for the expense of treatment. Employers are particularly willing to do this when they are involved in the treatment efforts or even when they are just kept abreast of the progress. This is not unique to addictions treatment, but seems to be more prevalent as employers begin to realize that with addictions, treatment often leads to full recovery, and the returning employee will once again be fully productive. Employers are also learning that it is less expensive to rehabilitate a good employee than to train a new one.

In order to maximize your ability to maintain control of the therapy and to successfully manage the review process, it is important to be aware that regardless of the criteria a managed care company uses, it is a system of review that is based on clinical criteria. Knowing DSM-IV (American Psychiatric Association 1994) will, at a minimum, give you access to the terminology and criteria similar to that used by all reviewers. Being concerned for the welfare of your patients means being their advocate. Your role is not to directly challenge the validity of the managed care review (this can be accomplished through your professional organization), but rather to present a thorough and complete picture of the salient issues affecting your patient's need for treatment. For example, giving the reviewer two symptoms of drug dependence when the DSM-IV requires at least three to substantiate the diagnosis may lead to a rejection even when the patient has a serious dependency. It is always best to deal with the reviewers in a professional way, avoiding the arguments that might arise from your zeal in defending the patient's need for treatment. Be familiar with your rights in the appeal process, and be prepared to use them to defend your decisions when necessary. Communicating clearly with the patient about the potential for insurance reimbursement denial, despite the seriousness of the pathology, and especially when there is some question as to the extent of the patient's insurance coverage, will help prevent direct conflicts with the patient.

Joining a variety of health maintenance organizations (HMOs) or preferred provider organizations (PPOs) may help to ensure a steady flow of patients, but this is not guaranteed, and the fee scale may be lower than your established and acceptable fee. Truly remaining a solo practitioner, on the other hand, may allow for greater independence in establishing your own fee scale, but it may place you in jeopardy of losing your referral base to physicians who are enrolled in those health care organizations. I have elected not to join HMOs or PPOs because I believe that having a solid referral base will protect me at least for a while. I closely observe the situation and recognize that I may have to join some managed care programs as the political climate changes, but, at present, I continue as a solo practitioner.

Confidence in your own self-worth is foremost in establishing a realistic fee schedule. Personal needs and professional criteria, such as advanced specialized training, years of clinical experience, academic rank, number of clinical hours to be filled, and the prevailing rate in your community, will all contribute to the establishment of your professional fee. Although I believe that the fee charged should be commensurate with the above factors, some flexibility should always exist to accommodate patients from various financial backgrounds.

Conclusion

Working with alcoholic and addicted patients is a rewarding experience. Although these patients are sometimes resistant to treatment, usually they are eager and appreciative to receive help. The clinical problems are both acute and chronic. Some problems require crisis intervention, and others need long-term supportive care. Psychodynamically oriented insight psychotherapy may be appropriate for those who stop drinking. Treatment is conducted in both an individual format and through social-support-system intervention. Patients do change and are quite appreciative of their improvement and the therapist's contribution. In all, alcoholism and addiction psychiatry offers the psychiatrist a range of opportunities in developing a clinical practice. It clearly lends itself well to a private practice model that can be both professionally and financially rewarding.

Reference

American Psychiatric Association: Diagnostic and Statistical Manual of Mental Disorders, 4th Edition. Washington, DC, American Psychiatric Association, 1994

Chapter 13

Practice of Geriatric Psychiatry

Judith H. W. Crossett, M.D., Ph.D.

I did not start medical school planning to be a geriatric psychiatrist—in fact, I had not thought of medicine at all until I was 29 years old, a mother, and halfway through a dissertation in English literature. I am the only physician in my family, although we have a strong family tradition of volunteer service in related fields, from the Red Cross Grey Ladies of World War II to the activists in hospice and Planned Parenthood today. In geriatric psychiatry, I have found a place to combine my love of medicine, my love of language, and my drive to be of use in my community. I am fortunate enough to have found a group of partners in private practice who enjoy and encourage diverse interests.

Much of medical education consists of learning to see what is in front of you, and to see it articulately so that you can describe it. We are taught that "if you didn't chart it, you didn't do it"; I would add that if you can't describe it, you don't see it. Most of my patients have a dementing illness; my job as a geriatric psychiatrist is to see these patients very clearly and to describe them so accurately that they can live as fully as possible. I also treat mood disorders, anxiety disorders, various psychotic syndromes, and an occasional case of alcoholism or posttraumatic stress disorder. Acutely psychotic schizophrenia, personality disorders, and eating disorders are very rare in my practice. I often tell my patients that my unofficial job description is first to keep them out of the hospital and, second, to keep them in their own homes, in their own community, as long as they want and we can make it work. Underlying this philosophy is an increasing belief in letting people live by their own choices, in their own style, as long as they are not in imminent danger or a threat to public health.

I particularly enjoy treating the problems of a patient who is confused, who requires not only all my powers of observation and thought, but also those of a team of allied professionals whom I summon, coordinate, and direct; I integrate their findings into the best plan I can offer to improve that patient's life. An inpatient geriatric psychiatry unit is my goal; at present, I have built a practice consisting of 70% hospital and nursing home work; the remainder is office-based outpatient psychiatry. The psychiatric and behavioral problems of dementia occupy most of my time. Over 90% of my patients are at least 60 years old; most are in their 70s and 80s. Although "my" team of nurses, social workers, occupational and recreational therapists, etc. also work with a general adult population on the same inpatient wards, they have developed some special programs and protocols for the older patients. I diagnose, direct, provide pharmacotherapy, talk to families, and constantly listen and educate.

I left academic medicine because I realized that what I enjoy most, and what I spend the majority of my time doing, is working with patients and their caregivers. My time reserved for writing grants was used up with patient care. I concluded that I would be happiest in a setting where I could devote all my time to patient care and where clinical practice is not just valued—it is the primary pursuit of everyone I work with. I miss the academic world where I enjoyed being a perpetual student; but realistically, the nonresearch clinician is outnumbered and not very highly valued in a university.

Training

I learned geriatric psychiatry on-the-job; by the time I finished my residency, I had acquired a master's degree in preventive medicine as part of a psychiatric epidemiology fellowship. I already had graduate degrees in English, and my daughter calculated that I had been in school or training for 36 years. It was time for my 25th high school reunion, not another fellowship. The residency program was very flexible; we could pursue any psychiatric interests, if we could persuade the chairman that we had data or at least a testable hypothesis. In my last 2 years, I "collected" elderly patients, read the geriatric and neurological literature, and took a moonlighting job in a geriatric outreach program. I was very fortunate in being chosen as an American Psychiatric Association/Burroughs-Wellcome Fellow, and thus spent 2 years on the American Psychiatric Association Council on Aging. By the time I was looking for my first "real" job, I had superb residency training in psychopharmacology, diagnosis, medical management, and neurology, as well as 2 years' experience weighted toward geriatric patients. Two years of geriatric psychiatry at a university-affiliated Veterans Administration hospital improved my skills, and I passed the examination for "Added Qualifications in Geriatric Psychiatry" without difficulty.

Today, I would consider a fellowship. First, the knowledge base in geriatric psychiatry has expanded rapidly and would be more difficult to pick up informally. Second, a fellowship is now prerequisite to eligibility for the added qualifications examination. Even in private practice, the certificate adds to my credibility, although like the general adult psychiatry board examination, it is not necessary for successful practice. Continuing education is essential; the American Association for Geriatric Psychiatry provides both that and a group where I am not one-of-a-kind.

Determining the Location and Type of Practice

We wanted to live in the upper Midwest because we like the climate and are at home here. As the single parent of a teenage girl, I wanted to live where my daughter could be safe and independent because I often would not be there to drive or supervise. It is also important to me to be in a community where I can have a network of friends, repairers, church, etc. I cannot depend on the kindness of strangers, and I know I often need support and the sense of belonging. I like having a college nearby, but I do not need a major metropolis.

I considered starting a solo geriatric psychiatry practice in Iowa City, but instead, I decided to live in Iowa City and join a psychiatric partnership in Cedar Rapids, 25 miles north. My reason for not going into solo practice was to avoid the burden of making all the business decisions myself (or paying someone and losing some control without losing the responsibility). I wanted to spare myself from questions such as "Where do you put your office? What furnishings? Who will clean it? Letterhead design? Which phone service? What style and size of telephone directory advertisement? Which receptionist and what other personnel do you hire?" I have a good friend who is the sole owner of a small business; thinking about his life helped me realize that I did not want to manage both a household and my own business.

By joining an established practice, I avoided setting up a business. As a partner, I share in business decisions, and I learn more each week about the decisions that must be made. How much of a raise and/or a bonus do we give each employee and with what consequences, not only financial, but also to the working relationships of the staff? If we do have a problem in the smooth running of the office staff, when do we let the staff solve it, when does the office manager step in, and when do we need to intervene?

Working in a partnership in which we make decisions by consensus, we can express different views—fiscal, social, political—from different philosophical bases and arrive at decisions that I think are remarkably good. I can see that my own liberal tendencies would leave me bankrupt providing benefits to my employees; now I can argue for greater generosity while being restrained from excess. The volume of our practice means we do not need to limit the number of Medicaid or Medicare patients we see; in solo practice, the lower reimbursement for these patients can make meeting expenses difficult.

Practice Description

The group I was invited to join consists of 7 active psychiatrists— 3 women and 4 men; 2 child and adolescent psychiatrists, 1 adult and adolescent psychiatrist, 3 general adult psychiatrists, and myself, a geriatric psychiatrist. We also have 2 part-time, semiretired psychiatrists; they both limit their time to outpatients—1 for children and the other for adults. We employ 2 psychologists, 1 for counseling, and 1 for neuropsychology; 2 social workers; a nurse; and an office staff of 11 (3 part-time). We have complementary, but not identical, styles of practice; we leave our patients in each others' care without concern when away. Most of us are primarily biologically oriented, although some have more psychodynamic training.

Each partner has developed special interests or tends to see certain types of patients. Although there is some banter about the type of patient one encounters when taking on a partner's patient load for a few days, we value the chance to keep up skills with young chronic schizophrenic patients, alcoholic patients, adolescents, personality disorder patients, eating disorder patients, children, and geriatric patients, as well as in general private practice adult psychiatry. We also provide psychiatric coverage by contract for a pain clinic and two county mental health centers in adjoining counties.

The other major reason to join a group, rather than a solo psychiatric practice, is the built-in sharing of nights, weekends, and vacations. I am fortunate to have a group with a casual approach; we are each responsible for our own patients from Monday morning through Saturday noon, and the remaining day and a half we rotate. A weekend on-call, covering two hospitals and seven psychiatrists' patients, can be exhausting—however, it only occurs once every 2 months. During the week, however, we can "sign out" to each other without prior arrangement for choir practice, a movie, a child's concert, or a ball game. I call the answering service: "This is Dr. Crossett; it's choir night, so I'm signing out to Dr. P." "He's already signed out to Dr. H., doctor." "Okay, sign us both out to him; I'll call you when I'm back." The only disadvantage is that my partners have some knowledge of my social life, particularly if I forget to sign in again. In fact, we rarely receive calls at night, and it is not burdensome.

Specifics of Geriatric Psychiatry

The burden in geriatric psychiatry falls most heavily on the nursing staff of the two hospitals where I have privileges. For psychiatric nurses whose role is often to give patients more one-to-one time talking about issues, feelings, stresses, and insights, caring for my patients is sometimes frustrating. Most of my hospitalized patients do not talk, or at least not coherently; they do not gain insight; they require a great deal of physical care.

A diagnosis with matching prescription, diet, and activity level are not adequate to care for my geriatric patients. For a cognitively impaired or physically frail patient, to help plan the best quality of life, we must also determine the stage of dementia, the specific strengths and deficits, and the activities and settings that will most benefit that person. I ask for a full neuropsychological battery on many patients, including Wechsler Adult Intelligence Scale—Revised (Wechsler 1981), Wechsler Memory Scale—Revised (Wechsler 1987), and Rey Auditory-Verbal Learning Test (Lezak 1983). The testing helps caregivers realize how serious the impairment is—or reassures them that there is no measurable decline or, perhaps, no further decline. Successful daily living, however, does not depend on formal intellectual and verbal skills. Ability to function in activities of daily living (e.g., dressing, bathing), the instrumental activities of daily living (using a telephone, a toaster), and following verbal, visual, or hand-on-hand cues are evaluated by occupational therapists. How many steps can the person remember at once? Will this person see the need to bathe or wash dishes without prompting? How successful will this person be in recognizing and solving an unexpected problem? Recreational therapists are needed also: how does this person tolerate a group, of what size, at what distance, and what kinds of interaction? Every encounter is therapeutic in psychiatry, but in geriatric psychiatry, every encounter is evaluative.

I enjoy the challenge of the evaluation, and I enjoy describing what my team has found. The goal is to find the setting in which that patient will function best by defining what functions remain and to find and explain treatment plans that caregivers can understand and use practically. This kind of evaluation requires that I listen to all the staff who help my patient. Their better understanding of what I am trying to do is an ongoing process; my rounds and staffings are always teaching rounds. My own learning is ongoing too; by listening to everyone else (at least as much as I talk, I hope), I learn about my patients and how to help them.

Of course, I also see outpatients in my office. Our partnership has just moved into its own building—enough offices and windows all around. Many of the features were designed with my geriatric patients (and building codes) in mind. The entrance is under a portico, with double doors and no steps. The restroom is fully wheelchair-accessible and immediately off the waiting room. My office is very close to the waiting room, and it is a "straight shot" to push a wheelchair into. We used a lot of wood and found a color scheme everyone is happy with (earth tones, restrained use of plum and teal). We compromised on the real versus artificial plant issue; we have many real plants, all donated from our own collections, and artificial ones in the offices of those few who prefer them. What we face now is paying for it.

Financial Issues

Geriatric psychiatry is not a very lucrative specialty. It is very demanding of time, but Medicare permits billing only for time you spend with the patient. As I practice, much of my time is spent with the team and with caregivers. The patient is there too, as often as possible, but

I dislike discussing a patient in the presence of others, particularly if the patient cannot understand us. Medicare reimbursement is significantly less than third-party reimbursement for equivalent services to those under age 65; less, in fact, than Title XIX (Medicaid) reimbursement in our area. I may bill my patients directly for "noncovered services," for deductibles, and for the relatively trivial difference between what Medicare allows and what Medicare will pay. I do regularly bill families who can afford it, and by prearrangement, for long family conferences, some of which take place over the telephone. I bill patients for telephone calls that are frequent, over 10 minutes, and replace office visits. I bill these at our current standard adult rate. Sometimes I am paid, and I virtually always "cure" inappropriate phone use. I do have some general adult patients—it is relaxing to treat a patient with standard adult major depression or panic disorder—and I do a little expert witness work and some medical directorship, all of which help to improve my income. But I do not think I could afford to practice geriatric psychiatry in the style I am accustomed to without the structure of my partnership.

The seven full partners in the group own an equal share of our capitalization. We equally share the building, furnishings, telephone and paging service, and all the intangibles that determine the net worth of the partnership. Each physician new to the group spends 1 year as an employee and then begins buying into the partnership. To buy in, some money is held from your biweekly draw until you have contributed enough for your share of the current capital worth. In effect, you buy your share on time but without interest payment. Once a fully paid-up partner, there is some return on the capital investment built into our financial structure.

At first, of course, a new physician has no money coming in—no patients have been seen, and no charges have been submitted to be divided into collections and receivables. During the first few months, your paycheck is really an advance from the partnership that you will have to pay back; given Medicare reimbursement, I needed to get patients quickly. People constantly call our office looking for a psychiatrist, or a new psychiatrist, or particularly for a woman psychiatrist. I had to be firm about not seeing nongeriatric patients or I would not have had a geriatric practice. My group and the two hospitals publicized my arrival and my special interest in geriatric psychiatry—and I never turn down a speaking engagement. Every time I go to medicine or neurology floors to do a consult, I talk with nursing staff, and as they learn what I can do, they often encourage other physicians to ask for my help.

Building the Practice

My partners gave me their geriatric emergency room (ER) admissions and ensured that I had extra ER call during the first few months (the ER call list is used for anyone who walks in needing a psychiatrist who does not already have one). A few patients were referred to the new geriatric specialist by other psychiatrists, but I learned that these were usually very difficult patients. Nursing home regulations, and my willingness to go to nursing homes, bring referrals. My practice built more slowly than a general adult practice might have, but I had all the work I wanted within 9 months. Now—3 years later—I am resisting the pressure to expand my hours until my daughter has finished high school.

Scheduling and Billing

We set our own schedule to see office and hospital patients. The usual pattern is to make hospital rounds in the morning and see office patients in the afternoon. Each physician decides whether to have evening and Saturday hours. I usually see new patients for an hour and returning patients for 15 to 30 minutes; the scheduling computer is very flexible. We each turn in our cards listing hospital patients seen and for what services each day; each office patient has a routing slip on which we circle the service and indicate diagnosis and interval to next appointment. All services are expressed in units of 15 minutes: a two-unit visit is 16 to 30 minutes long. We use codes for medical psychotherapy, hospital care, consultation, admission history and physical examination, and electroconvulsive therapy (ECT). Two staff members convert these data into computer data so that bills are sent to third parties (often electronically filed), each physician is correctly credited with the charges billed, and then the amount is collected from those charges. The percentage of charges actually collected varies; mine, based on the Medicare structure, run lower than average for the group. We do accept assignment, and we participate in two or three managed health care plans, but most geriatric patients are retired and not part of these employment-based plans.

From the total collection for the group, we pay our overhead: employee costs, building costs, telephones, advertising, and malpractice insurance. In general, anything we all use is considered overhead paid by the group. Professional memberships, however, are paid individually. An equal percentage is taken from each partner's collections for overhead. Thus, the partners with the largest practices pay higher absolute amounts toward overhead, and practices that are smaller because of reimbursement patterns or a choice to work fewer hours pay less—but we all pay the same percentage of our income toward expenses. We have no minimum expectation for earnings. In effect, this system (which was established when the partnership was set up and long before I joined) makes it possible for me to do the work I love, because my partners are subsidizing my overhead. I may take less of the typists' time (fewer notes for fewer patients) but not, I suspect, significantly less space, telephone use, or overall staff time.

My own practice consists of hospital rounds in the morning, which I do at a leisurely pace unless I have more than 6 hospitalized patients. I have had up to 12 at once; fortunately I had a family practice geriatric fellow with me that month. I usually have 1 or 2 inpatients undergoing ECT treatment (and occasionally do series for other psychiatrists who choose not to do their own ECT). I also have a few elderly patients on outpatient maintenance ECT. I often have patients to consult on from medicine, neurology, orthopedics, and the skilled nursing units. Once a week, I meet briefly with the staff from each psychiatric unit to discuss overall progress and treatment plans for each of my patients— although in effect I talk to most of them every day.

Afternoons I keep varied. I spend two afternoons each month as medical director for two nursing homes, consulting about overall care plans and policies and helping them meet nursing home regulations on restraints and psychopharmacological agents. One afternoon each week I see individual patients in nursing homes in three counties. Most of these are one-time consultations with occasional follow-up visits. The allowable charge for a consultation—if the attending physician's order for the consultation is on the chart—subsidizes the return visits, for which I seldom bill because the reimbursement is so low. The remaining afternoons I see patients in my office.

I choose not to work evenings and Saturdays in the office, and I also choose to spend a good deal of essentially unbillable time talking with nursing staff and caregivers. When my daughter starts college,

I will have less reason to preserve my time at home and may need to reduce the time I spend in nursing homes. I will miss the luxury of educating both myself and others, but tuition bills will probably not respect the values of my current style. I do not have late appointments on Wednesday afternoons so that I can attend choir practice, and I will continue that even when I make other shifts in my time allocation.

Geriatric Practice Difficulties

I have mentioned third-party oversight and nursing home regulations in passing; they do cause some particular difficulties for geriatric practice. To hospitalize a patient, I do not need to "precertify" the need for admission as long as Medicare is the primary payer. I do need to be careful that my charges reflect time spent with the patient, and, of course, I do not charge "medical psychotherapy" for patients with dementia.

Length of stay creates most of my problems. I will not discharge a patient for whom I do not believe we have a workable discharge plan and setting. Sometimes nursing homes are reluctant to readmit a patient with behavior problems even when I believe the problem is managed. The hospital now requires as a condition for admission a letter from the facility administrator that the patient will be reaccepted without quali-fication. Most nursing homes have always reaccepted their own resi-dents; a few homes have learned that the hospital cannot help them if they burden the hospital with difficult patients who stay long. Medicaid (Title XIX) will only pay to hold a bed for a nursing home resident for 10 days; families often cannot pay for additional days to hold the bed. I try to plan in advance the treatment I will offer the 10-day patients and return them promptly with at least some problems defined and allevi-ated. When we need more time, we ask that the nursing home put the patient at the top of the waiting list; we do not expect nursing homes to subsidize empty beds. For all my patients, Utilization Review oversees whether the patient continues to improve or that I continue to evaluate and try new treatments to justify continued stay. I very rarely need to call external reviewers myself, and third-party oversight has not yet prevented me from giving the care I believe appropriate in the hospital.

In nursing homes, however, oversight makes psychiatric care very difficult. Nursing homes have always had a high percentage of resi-dents with psychiatric symptoms and illness. Current regulations under

OBRA (Omnibus Budget Reconciliation Act) intend to ensure appropriate care for each resident in the least restrictive manner and emphasize the resident's rights. In practice, the interpretive guidelines and particular state reviewers who monitor nursing home practices make provision of psychiatric medication very difficult. Medications and even physical restraints are allowed under these regulations, but their use requires documentation by the physician of diagnosis, efficacy, and side effects and copious documentation from the facility. Efforts are to be made to reduce medications and restraints at regular intervals, and the doctor's order is never sufficient justification. Much of my practice consists of providing the appropriate diagnoses and rationale for using psychotropic medications and continuing the doses. Sometimes I feel as if I am treating charts and reviewers, but for all the irritation of the paperwork, the observations of these patients that must be made for good nursing care, diagnosis, and medication review are simply part of good medical practice.

Political Issues and Educational Activities

Nursing home issues do provide an opportunity for some political activism, which I also enjoy. One version of the OBRA implementation in the federal register required that an independent geriatric psychiatrist or geriatric internist annually review all psychotropic use by each nursing home patient. In this relatively rural state, we have some board-certified geriatric internists, but to the best of my knowledge, I am the only psychiatrist with a certificate of added qualifications in geriatric psychiatry. I wrote to and called some agencies concerned with the rules and was told my input helped modify that rule—I am flattered, but cannot spend all my time reviewing medications.

My presence as the only geriatric psychiatrist in the state does bring elderly patients in from a wider area than my partnership normally serves. I am occasionally called on for a newspaper story or a television spot when Alzheimer's disease is in the news, and I often speak at continuing education conferences for family practice, nurses, etc. All of these activities help educate the public and the profession about the possibilities of help from geriatric psychiatry, and they do help bring new patients of all ages to our practice.

I often speak without a fee, particularly for service organizations, the Alzheimer's Association, or for small nursing homes in the immediate area. Sponsoring educational institutions usually offer expenses and honoraria from $50 to a few hundred dollars; educational programs ultimately sponsored by pharmaceutical companies have less constrained budgets and will have slides made, etc. I keep expense money; any honoraria are paid into the partnership as part of my collections.

I enjoy public speaking; it is another way to help educate more people about what psychiatry can do. I went through high school and college with the civil rights movement; now I combat prejudices and attitudes about aging and the aging mind: "What can you do for these old people, anyway?," "Of course he (or she) is senile, after all, he's ___ (fill in any age)." I have been fortunate to have parents and grandparents who remained curious, interested in the world, and without time to do all they wished despite physical frailty until they died. Perhaps, like teaching or ministry, geriatric psychiatry requires a commitment and love of the work that overrides the financial limitations. I am extraordinarily fortunate to be able to live where I choose, to have colleagues who value and support what I do, and to do the work I love.

References

Lezak M: Rey Auditory-Verbal Learning Test, in Neuropsychological Assessment, 2nd Edition. New York, Oxford, 1983

Wechsler D: Wechsler Adult Intelligence Scale—Revised. San Antonio, TX, Psychological Corporation, 1981

Wechsler D: Wechsler Memory Scale—Revised. San Antonio, TX, Psychological Corporation, 1987

Chapter 14

Forensic Psychiatric Practice

Kenneth J. Weiss, M.D.

*F*orensic or legal psychiatry is the application of psychiatric principles, methods, and knowledge to legal questions that require illumination by an expert. Expert testimony, in turn, is required by courts when the knowledge or experience of the trier of fact (judge or jury) is not sufficient to permit an unaided decision. Testimony is often needed in a wide variety of situations: psychiatric injuries, disability, criminal responsibility, criminal or civil competency matters, dangerousness, domestic disputes, and civil rights. Forensic practice spans both private and public-sector activities. Branches of forensic psychiatry found in the public sector are correctional psychiatry (jails or prisons), court clinics, and the institutional care of the "criminally insane" or intractably dangerous. Some of these areas can be integrated into a private practice by way of a contract with the county or state.

There are nearly 300 diplomats of the American Board of Forensic Psychiatry and about 1,500 members of the American Academy of Psychiatry and the Law (AAPL), but several thousand members of the American Psychiatric Association have identified themselves as devoting a portion of their time to forensic matters. As the mounting pressure against traditional private practice continues to erode the role of psychiatry in some clinical areas, the practice of forensic psychiatry may become a potential refuge for clinicians. In this chapter, I will outline the structure of the private practice of forensic psychiatry, including aspects of professional identity, career satisfaction, time management, and financial rewards.

Role and Identity Issues

There are many possible portals of entry into forensic practice. Residents are often intrigued by the introduction of psychiatry into courtroom drama. Psychiatrists in practice may be asked to participate in a case and find it rewarding. Others have had a long-standing interest in the law, but chose a career in medicine. In any case, the practitioner may have to make adjustments in practice style and self-image.

My entry point into forensic practice came early in my career, after having been immersed in community psychiatry after residency training. I was encouraged by an attorney friend to try my hand at participating in a criminal case, a homicide, for the public defender. At this point, I was already in an academic career. I had little coaching from the public defender and no experience with testimony outside of commitment hearings. On cross-examination, I was asked for the defendant's diagnosis. DSM-III (American Psychiatric Association 1980) had just been published, and not wanting to be pushed around by the prosecutor, I asserted that the defendant had a "mental disorder," rejecting the terminology "mental disease." To my chagrin, my assertiveness brought the entire proceeding to a screeching halt; the jury was unseated, and the attorneys met with the judge in chambers. I stayed—uncomfortably—on the witness stand. A kindly senior trial attorney sidled over to me and said, sotto voce, "You have to say mental disease or you can't testify." Soon enough, the conference was over, and with the jury back in the room, the judge turned to me and asked, "Doctor, is it your testimony that the defendant had a mental disease at the time of the homicide?" I reasoned that "Yes, Your Honor" might be a good response. The rest of the testimony was uneventful, and the defense lost its case. Several things were apparent to me afterward: I enjoyed the lively exchange of courtroom drama. I had a chance to educate citizens about the effects of mental illness on behavior. And I had much to learn about this strange world of the law, where one word can make a difference.

Gradually, over the years, including accepting diverse cases, some fellowship training, and self-directed study, I felt ready to take forensic psychiatry seriously. Then, when I began to read and study for my forensic board examination, I realized how rich the literature and traditions of the field were. After passing the examinations, I focused on quality: adhering to principles of practice, managing time and money, and becoming more involved in my peer-group activities. I have been able to integrate a wide-ranging forensic practice with teaching and a principally psychopharmacological ambulatory practice. Although my affiliation is with a private sector university hospital, the forensic practice is run on a private practice model. My patients know that, at times, I may be called into court, and they have been very understanding and rarely mistreated.

Professional Identity

The most fundamental characteristic of forensic practice is that it is the practice of psychiatry, not law, law enforcement, or jurisprudence, as fascinating as they may be in their own right. The quality basis for forensic psychiatry is excellence in general psychiatry, adult or child/family. The legal and justice systems are extremely complex and tend to be alien with respect to the environment in which physicians are accustomed to operating. Lawyers feel the same way about medicine, too, exemplified by the archaic term for an expert witness: *alienist*.

Any of us who have been summoned to court, stumbled into a matter under litigation, or been identified as a defendant can attest that few experiences in practice are as likely to raise our blood pressure and cause sleepless nights. Among psychiatrists in general there appears to be a fear, bordering on contempt, of the legal world. There is an asymmetry between physicians and attorneys: they're always doing things to us, whereas we seem helpless to influence them. Small wonder, given that legislators and judges tend to be legal professionals first. Dealing effectively with our natural reticence would be a sine qua non of a successful forensic practice.

One of the most difficult tasks in the beginning of forensic practice is to stay focused on professional identity. Suddenly, you're a "defense expert" or "witness for the prosecution," immediately identified with a cause that you had no role in creating nor interest in the outcome. Although no special knowledge and skills may be necessary to be a successful expert witness, one must always keep in mind not to stray from the principles and practice of psychiatry. When in doubt, repeat this to yourself as if a mantra: "I'm a psychiatrist." The implication of this centering exercise is the realization that you know more about your subject than anyone else in the courtroom, and no one can take that away from you. Even the dreaded "battle of experts" is somewhat fictional: it is not a face-to-face debate to determine whether another doctor is smarter than you.

We are accustomed to treating patients. We have traditionally held the revered position as healers, forming dyadic relationships with our customers to benefit their health. It is not so simple in private forensic practice. We see a major permutation of the health care model: the attorney, court, or agency is our client (from a business perspective), and a plaintiff, defendant, or petitioner is the subject of the psychiatric inquiry. Sometimes we do not even see "patients," when the subject of the inquiry is a deceased patient or an allegedly incompetent deceased testator. An attorney will often ask us to derive an opinion about another professional's quality of care or a person's state of mind solely on the basis of documents. In the beginning, this may give rise to anomie in the psychiatrist, who is accustomed to a medical end. By contrast, the legal end—justice—is always serving someone else's goals, and we are instruments to those ends.

If patients are not our employers, for whom are we working? Judges ask us to help them seek the truth; prosecutors want us to help them lock up—or kill—a defendant; the defendants' lawyers use us to keep those same citizens out of prison; civil rights advocates ask us to secure liberty for citizens, sometimes sacrificing treatment; and civil lawyers are in the business to make money for their clients or to minimize the damages. The potential forensic professional will have to make perceptual adjustments to live peaceably with this model.

Anyone possessing knowledge, training, education, or experience in an area that a court is addressing can be qualified to give expert testimony. Usually, the testimony is preceded by a written report, submitted to the lawyer who hired you, and shared with the other side (the process of discovery). This is another strange twist in the practice style, because your report becomes, literally, a public document. Often, the case never goes to trial, and it is on the strength of your written work that cases are won or lost. Therefore, a relative aptitude with words, and the potential to back them up in speech, are important ingredients for the potential forensic psychiatrist.

If any professional can be an expert witness, how does the judge or jury find "facts" amid conflicting testimony? This is another situation with which the practitioner must reconcile with standard medical practice. Only one side can win, and the trier of fact will be as likely as not to find for the other side. This does not mean you were wrong on your own terms, rather that another opinion carried the day on that occasion. Therefore, forensic practice includes not overinvesting ego in the outcome of cases. Career satisfaction here must reside in presenting quality written and oral work and on trying to prevail without over-identifying with a cause. Once you become accustomed to it, it is even possible to enjoy the experience of testimony. A gladiatorial trait may be useful for experts, but leave the real carnage to the lawyers.

Education and Training

Although I have said that anyone with relevant experience can be an expert, special training is necessary to be a competent forensic psychiatrist. It is not simply a matter of credentials in the courtroom, but one of learning a new way to practice under supervision. The following models of postgraduate education are options.

- *Fellowship:* There are over 30 fellowship programs in forensic psychiatry, mostly at the fifth to sixth postgraduate year (PGY-V to VI) level. There is an accreditation board and process for fellowships. It is unsettled at this time what the significance of fellowship accreditation will be for eligibility to sit for the added-qualifications examination of the American Board of Psychiatry and Neurology (ABPN). A listing of fellowship programs can be obtained from the AAPL's executive office in Connecticut or at its display at the American Psychiatric Association's annual meeting. For the psychiatrist or resident with definite inclinations toward a forensic career, fellowship training of at least a year is highly recommended. The advantages are continuous and high-quality supervision, entry into the subspecialty network, and an opportunity for in-depth reading and research.
- *Apprenticeship:* Although it is difficult to arrange, the practicing psychiatrist who cannot enter a fellowship program may consider obtaining supervision from an established forensic practitioner. The essential elements of such a program would be mutual observation and discussion of cases, review of the trainee's written work product and testimony, and a reading program.
- *Self-directed study:* Perhaps, by default, the most common educational route is also the riskiest, because of the potential for unproductive habits to develop. At the least, the practitioner should attempt to obtain some supervision of written work and to undertake a structured

reading program. There are several excellent texts on forensic psychiatry. Just as important are landmark legal cases, board review courses, and audiotapes and other educational materials available through the AAPL. These efforts should be supplemented by continuing education, as described below.

Entering the Field

Too few psychiatrists are willing to take forensic cases. Once you do, success is not automatic. It depends on both your clinical skill and your ability to develop a reputation for quality among colleagues and attorneys.

Practice Development

Developing and maintaining a forensic psychiatric practice is a process similar to that in clinical private practice: making appropriate contacts, providing high quality and timely work products, and demonstrating reliability over time. This does not mean you have to win cases. That is the advocate's job. Your product is credibility and integrity: representing psychiatry and its knowledge and methods, without overidentifying with a legal issue. A few elements of practice development are noteworthy.

- *Reputation:* Although lawyers are usually driven by habit to call experts they believe are reliable (for an honest opinion, not a particular opinion), they may also look for a fresh face. It is not uncommon for lawyers to call practitioners who are well reputed in the community. Because most of our colleagues want nothing to do with legal matters, it is wise for the budding forensic professional to advise colleagues to send over inquiries.

  There is usually no analogy in forensic practice to applying for medical staff privileges at a hospital. The closest thing would be to volunteer to be on a panel of experts for assignment at a court clinic. This is a wise choice, because you may be able to do evaluations and have your work product circulated, and, more important, you may appear in court, where you will get experience and exposure. The exposure will be to lawyers on both sides, as well as to the judge or any other attorneys who may be in the courtroom. If you perform credibly, such exposure may open the door for opportunities, because the most common referral source is word-of-mouth by the lawyers' networks.

- *Public relations:*   There are more aggressive approaches to practice development, which in my experience, are secondary to reputation and exposure. These include writing an article about a psychiatric topic for a law magazine; giving a speech on a psychiatric topic to a local bar association; giving interviews to newspapers or other media about social or psychiatric topics; and taking out advertising space in a law publication or forensic services clearinghouse. In theory, the least credible of these is advertising. I have heard both sides of the story: referrals coming from advertisements and lawyers who say they would never use an expert who advertises.

- *Forensic professionals' groups:*   Some cities have organizations dedicated to promoting services to the legal profession. One group I was a member of included experts in psychology, jury selection, accident reconstruction, firearms, hypnosis, economics, and engineering. There is a noncompetitive quid pro quo implied when cross-referrals are made among disciplines. More formally, two important national organizations are worth joining. The AAPL is the best-known forensic psychiatry group. Becoming an active member of AAPL can be extremely valuable in establishing a forensic practice. The second is the American Academy of Forensic Sciences, which has a section on behavioral sciences, emphasizing psychiatry. Both organizations have outstanding annual meetings and publications in addition to the opportunity to meet the right people.

Collegial Support

Many forensic psychiatrists consider themselves "lone wolves," in the sense that much of the work is done outside of organized psychiatry. Although this is not very different from solo practice, there is a dimension of alienation, because your contacts are not doctors and patients, but criminals, litigants, and legal professionals. You may even start speaking and thinking like a lawyer. I see nothing wrong with making empathic bonds to the field of law, but it must be tempered by a more fundamental connection to your roots in psychiatry. For reasons given above, participation in a forensic organization (e.g., AAPL) can be a critical factor in both developing the practice and maintaining a sense of identity. In addition to a superb educational format, as with any peer group, the very presence of other professionals struggling with the same issues is tremendously reassuring and can make the difference in your ability to persevere.

Personal Development

In the practice of law, as well as in psychiatry, some practitioners (e.g., the litigators) have substantial forensic skills, whereas others prefer to bury their noses in paper, equally useful but less personally challenging. Most of us find it challenging to interact with patients in the pursuit of medical goals. When lawyers evaluate us as potential experts, they need to satisfy themselves that we can think, write, speak, and be persuasive and credible in the service of their legal goals. Although there are no absolute minimum requirements for the qualities of experts, the following are suggestions.

Credentials. Attorneys who hire experts like to emphasize impressive-sounding credentials, such as academic appointments, board certifications, publications, and honors. It is difficult to know whether judges and juries pay attention to paper credentials, or whether they are more likely to listen to someone who looks convincing and credible. At a minimum, the expert witness should be certified by the ABPN. Additional certification, for example, by the American Board of Forensic Psychiatry (the old boards) or ABPN's added qualifications in forensic psychiatry (the new boards), adds weight to credentials but does not permit the expert witness to testify differently.

Any medical school faculty appointment is helpful, and, in my experience, not much is made of distinctions between full-time academics and volunteer faculty. During the qualifications phase of your testimony, the attorney proffering your testimony will ask you to speak at length about your experiences and accomplishments. The opposing attorney, through the process of voir dire, will be able to challenge your admissibility as an expert, although, in practice, a successful challenge on credentials is virtually impossible. At other times, the opposing counsel will stipulate to your qualifications, often in an attempt to preempt your telling the jury about yourself. I would take this as a compliment. Sometimes you are allowed to speak anyway.

The main point of presenting credentials is to impress on the judge or jury the relevance of your training and experience to the question before the court. If you are an experienced clinician who has seen hundreds of patients with schizophrenia, you are in a position to educate the court about this disease and its likely effects on a person's behavior. This is the time to remind yourself that you really are an expert, perhaps not the world's authority on a subject within psychiatry, but someone who, by the legal definition, is in a position to educate the court. If you have written something on the subject, so much the better. Caution: you may be cross-examined on something you have written or even testified about in another case.

Teaching ability. Sometimes good clinical psychiatrists find their way into the courtroom, but do not succeed as forensic professionals. The reason is that forensic psychiatry is, to some degree, a performing art. You do not learn this in the consultation room. The purpose of expert testimony is to educate the trier of fact. How you go about this process is a matter of style, technique, and experience. Direct testimony should be considered a classroom experience, in which the jurors or judge are the students. The difference is that the question-and-answer period will be in the form of cross-examination, often intended to make you look less knowledgeable or at least incorrect. You must also keep in mind that the jury has heard or will hear a different point of view from the opposing expert. This fact should not shake your self-confidence, as long as you have enough psychiatric data to support your position.

Unlike legal education, where mock trials are a behavioral rehearsal, psychiatric education does little to prepare us for giving testimony. Any background in either public speaking or classroom education is a good place to start. The hopeful forensic expert will take opportunities to give lectures on clinical topics that can be used in the courtroom as well. Courses on testimony are available through the American Psychiatric Association and the AAPL.

Confidence versus arrogance. The expert witness should have confidence in the psychiatric basis for the opinions expressed. The expert does not have to be absolutely right or to go out on a limb to overstate an opinion. It may be comforting to know that expert opinions, with few exceptions, are expressed to a degree of proof known as reasonable medical certainty. This means that an inference has been drawn between the psychiatric data and the legal question that makes it more likely than not that a legal standard has been met—that is, 51% probable. For example, you may testify that it is reasonably certain that a defendant does not possess the requisite capacity to stand trial. The fact that there may be as much as 49% uncertainty is not your problem; it is the judge's or jury's. Trying to overstate your opinion is gratuitous and comes across as arrogant, an unfortunate quality for a forensic expert. The opposing expert, remember, may also have confidence but be more likable by the jury.

Credibility.   Although you may think the inherent truth in your opinion will be obvious to anyone, reading over the transcript of your testimony can be a sobering experience. It is not difficult for your testimony to be admissible, but how much weight it is given is a function of credibility. Sometimes, for example, we are asked to present psychiatric information that is counterintuitive; for example, a criminal defendant knew what he was doing but didn't know it was wrong because of a delusion. The psychiatric expert must become accustomed to adjusting vocabulary and concepts to the courtroom. The use of overly abstract concepts, jargon, and "high falutin" language generally work against you. Credibility, then, is a function of presentation style and ability to render your material intuitively plausible. This requires practice. Neat appearance and a serious (not pompous) manner are also important qualities.

Practice Management

The practitioner's ability to manage time and money is a generic skill. As a result of the peculiarities of forensic practice, the following considerations should be taken into account when entering the subspecialty.

* *Time commitment:*   No absolute minimum time requirement must be devoted to forensic activities. Few practitioners are in the exclusive private practice of forensic psychiatry. However, one should consult the ABPN for time and duration requirements as they pertain to sitting for the added qualifications examination. It is not difficult for the average private practitioner, who has pieced together several elements of a practice, to include an occasional legal matter, such as examining

a litigant in a personal injury case. I do not recommend dabbling in the criminal area, because more knowledge of the law is required, and it is more likely that testimony will be required. For child psychiatrists, however, the possibility of being drawn into a legal matter is stronger, because of involvement with child abuse and child custody matters. I strongly encourage child- and family-oriented practitioners to become familiar with local statutes and to seek advice on the preparation of forensic reports and delivering live testimony.

• *Maintaining a treatment practice:* For practitioners who wish to have a forensic-oriented practice, it is possible to integrate forensic and nonforensic activities. For reasons of credibility, maintaining a treatment practice is useful. I have become the county jail psychiatrist, which is essentially a community mental health position, but the patients/inmates have no trouble conforming to my schedule. I maintain a practice of evaluation and treatment of sick persons while having the flexibility to negotiate court appearances and travel for evaluations. A few forensic psychiatrists have given up the treatment portion of the practice. Again, because of credibility (juries like real doctors), this is not recommended until the forensic practice is well established, and then only with reservations.

• *Combining forensic with other forms of private practice:* This is viable, depending on the practitioner's organizational skills. It works least well with a large solo practice and best with an inpatient/consultation style, in which you are not locked into office hours.

Time Management

As a rule, forensic work can play havoc with a psychiatrist's schedule. It is one thing to schedule appointments for forensic evaluations, but another to have to negotiate times for a deposition, or worse, to rely on the organization of the courts to block out time for your testimony. If you primarily review documents for civil matters, it is unlikely that you will go to court. However, the practice style of the full-range forensic professional often must make allowances for testimony at criminal hearings and trials. Unfortunately, as anyone involved in courts knows, trials are continued or postponed, the trial before yours runs late, judges get sick and take vacations, and you may have something else pressing.

One solution is to leave blocks of time in your schedule to shift activities around. Most of us will be able to fill a half day of canceled testimony with "billable hours" of document review, report writing, or visiting a defendant in jail. This style is difficult to reconcile with full-time private practice, unless it includes blocks of time used for inpatient rounds or consultations. It is easy to envision the embarrassment of having to move the appointments of private outpatients on a regular basis. Consequently, many dedicated forensic psychiatrists have limited office hours, which, for negotiating with attorneys, are inviolable.

Time is money. No lawyer will take issue with that. Therefore, the forensic professional should be able to charge for time used in ways different from sessions with patients. These include travel, paperwork, telephone calls, conferences, and time blocked out for testimony (whether or not you actually testify). Developing a forensic practice includes being entitled to compensation for your time, in the performance of activities that many of your colleagues eschew. Remember to establish ground rules in the beginning of the case: who is paying for what, how much, and when your time is retained. Most of the time, this leads to a happy conclusion.

Financial Arrangements

Because good forensic professionals are scarce, and the subspecialty is not dominated by medical third parties, the practitioner may have the advantage of earning good fees for service. Most experts agree that fees for forensic services can exceed those for clinical services. The overall profitability of forensic practice is a function of time management, volume, and referrals, as in ordinary private practice. The following are distinguishing features of forensic psychiatric practice.

* *Billable hours:*   If you have ever hired a lawyer, you have noticed that he or she is not shy about billing for any time or effort related to your case, as well as the services of others and incidental expenses. This is not meant as criticism, and, in fact, most dedicated forensic practitioners have adopted a similar model. There is no reason to be shy about charging for effort, whether it is reviewing documents, telephone conferences, or sitting in court waiting to be called to the witness stand. Many practitioners have different rates for various services, usually higher for live appearances than for paperwork. The practitioner must become accustomed to this, because billing for paperwork and incidental time for clinical services is only a fantasy in ordinary practice.

• *Retainer fees:* You may also notice that lawyers often get money "up front" in the form of a retainer fee. The reason for this is obvious; they cannot ensure the outcome of the case, and a losing client may not be disposed to paying a bill after the trial. Many forensic psychiatrists have also adopted the retainer fee as a standard arrangement. This is not unethical, and it is a good way to ease your mind as you proceed with a case. The theory is that an expert should be paid in advance so that there is no perceived threat on the expert's part that payment will be contingent on the quality of the testimony or on the outcome of the case. Incidentally, arranging for a contingency fee (i.e., a fee based on the outcome of the case) is unethical in psychiatry. At times, you may agree to defer your fee, but the amount must be set in advance.

The rules about asking for retainer fees are, whenever possible, obtain a retainer when a civil plaintiff's attorney (e.g., medical malpractice, personal injury) asks you to look at a case, or when a criminal defendant's attorney asks you to examine the client. In each case, explicitly state that the acceptance of the fee is not an indication that you will find something helpful. You must maintain independence of thought. When dealing with civil matters on the defense side, criminal prosecution cases, or public sector matters (e.g., public defenders, courts, advocates), it may not be possible to secure a retainer fee. However, have an agreement—written is best—about your fee schedule and an estimate of charges.

Problem Areas

If forensic psychiatry were as wonderful as I believe it is, why doesn't everyone do it? Many reasons can be inferred from the discussion thus far. I present the following points to identify the negative side of forensic practice.

• *Loss of clinical continuity:* By nature, and self-selection for our profession, psychiatrists are interested in helping patients improve. We do this over time, using various therapies. In most forensic work (the exception being correctional venues) we cannot fall back on our traditional identity as healers. To keep the forensic professional centered on psychiatry, and to enhance credibility in the courtroom, it is important to maintain a clinical practice. Legal professionals want to recognize that you are really a physician, someone who can also educate and relate to the law. Although the forensic psychiatrist deals with cases, it is not the same hands-on experience as with treatment. In addition, there is little control over the outcome of the legal matter, regardless of how good a physician one may be. Another peculiarity is that many civil cases lie dormant for years. A case may then come to trial, requiring expert testimony, after the expert has all but forgotten the details.

- *Overidentification with lawyers:* There is no reason that psychiatrists cannot be enamored of the law and its methods. Some forensic psychiatrists attend law school, although it is doubtful that this would improve performance as a psychiatrist. If you are attracted to the practice of law or even law enforcement, be clear that these are different from forensic psychiatry, which seeks only to apply a branch of medicine to legal settings. Becoming obsessed with winning and losing or with specific causes tends to diminish your potency as a witness. This does not mean that you must not align yourself with worthwhile advocacy causes, but that neutrality and credibility are more fundamental to sustaining a private forensic practice. Loss of perspective will lead to frustration and professional burnout.

- *Being used:* When you are in the legal universe you are still practicing psychiatry, but not as an autonomous practitioner. Your services are being employed as a means to a legal end. Although psychiatrists in this subspecialty gain comfort with the concept, many bristle in the face of perceived exploitation. This fact of forensic life is usually tolerable, more so by paying attention to the fundamental rule of maintaining professional identity across settings.

- *Being cast as a hired gun:* It is one thing to be paid for work that includes expressing opinions and another to have an opinion for hire. Some critics of forensic work blur that distinction and, sadly, so do some practitioners. Ethically, we are bound to honesty in our professional opinions. We should avoid temptation to stretch our opinions to fit the procrustean bed of legal standards or ends. Nevertheless, forensic psychiatrists may be the object of scorn from colleagues and popular opinion. Expert witnesses, in general, are ridiculed as purveyors of "junk science" and practitioners of professional prostitution. It helps to have a thick skin about these things and to remain centered on quality. If you are asked to do something questionable or beyond your ability, just say "no." You thereby retain self-respect and, at best, the respect of the attorney who must depend on your credibility.

Conclusion

For me, forensic psychiatric practice has been rewarding on many levels. I use all of my general psychiatric knowledge and analytic skills, I participate in settings that would be closed to me otherwise, I am rewarded reasonably for my time, I can expand my teaching and public speaking skills, and I commune with an exceptional peer group. I also find it interesting to try to navigate the communication barriers with the legal profession, to translate psychiatric knowledge into admissible opinions, and to deal with, not only angry litigants, but murderers and other severely disturbed individuals who may have mental disorders. It is in these areas, distinguishing injury from opportunism and sick from bad, that the forensic psychiatrist often dwells. Rewards lie in being helpful to the justice system and in applying psychiatric knowledge in a way that enhances the respectability of psychiatry as a whole.

Reference

American Psychiatric Association: Diagnostic and Statistical Manual of Mental Disorders, 3rd Edition. Washington, DC, American Psychiatric Association, 1980

Afterword

Successful Psychiatric Practice in the Present and Future

Edward K. Silberman, M.D.

*D*espite predictions of its impending death, private practice remains the mode of choice of the majority of psychiatrists graduating from American residency programs (Anonymous 1993, Born 1992). Although the financial advantages of private practice may have diminished over the past decade, its potential for autonomy, flexibility, and creativity continue to be very alluring to graduating residents. The current and future challenges of practicing psychiatrists are to maintain these values and to preserve the individuality and intimacy in the doctor-patient relationship that have been the traditional hallmarks of psychiatric practice.

The narratives in this book describe how a wide range of practices of various types and in various settings can be professionally rich and rewarding. Our definition of success encompasses not only financial viability, but the ability to shape a practice according to one's own interests and to treat patients according to one's own best judgment. This does not mean that it is possible to practice without making compromises or accepting financial and administrative constraints. It does mean that psychiatrists can practice in the current climate without abandoning their essential goals and integrity.

Although the authors describe a great diversity of practices and personal preferences, they are in considerable agreement about the essentials of success. The following elements appear repeatedly in their recommendations:

- *Clarity of purpose*—Knowing what you want is an essential prerequisite for attaining it. A clearly defined professional focus influences patient selection, communication with potential referring sources, continuing educational activities, and allocation of time. In contrast, vagueness about goals leads to inefficient use of time, the need for repeated back-tracking, and a disorganized career plan.

- *Professional competence*—Competition and professional ethics demand that you be as well trained as possible in your area of practice. Success of your practice requires that your patients feel well served and convey this to their referring doctors and other potential patients. Good training can be acquired on the job as well as through formal subspecialty programs, but you must remain actively involved in continuing education activities throughout your career.

- *Personal conviction*—You must believe in your method of treatment and your skill in delivering it in order to instill confidence in your patients and referring sources. Especially if you are recommending treatments such as psychoanalysis or long-term psychotherapy, which require considerable commitments of time and money from the patient, your personal conviction may determine whether your practice is viable.

- *Involvement in the medical community*—Psychiatrists cannot function in isolation from the rest of the medical community. To be successful in practice, other physicians must know who you are and what you do. They must know that you are available to help them with their clinical problems and referrals and that you are also a referral source for them. So that other physicians identify with you, you must work with them on common concerns through committees and organizations, and you must speak a language they can understand. You must also participate actively in psychiatric organizations to advocate for your professional concerns, pursue continuing education, and establish a professional support network.

- *Availability*—Creating easy access to your services is cited repeatedly as a cornerstone of building a practice. Seeing patients promptly and being willing to take on all or almost all referrals (including those who may not be able to pay your full fee) is essential, especially in the early stages of a practice. The ability to be highly selective may be an end goal for practitioners, but it cannot be an initial strategy.

- *Specialization*—Even general psychiatry practitioners benefit from having areas of special clinical interest and skill. Such areas help to focus your identity in the minds of referrers and enhance your own professional satisfaction.

- *Flexibility*—Although it is important to develop and maintain your own standards of treatment, success in the current period of change necessitates a flexible, open-minded approach to different modes of treatment and modes of practice. The practitioner who is willing to try both short- and long-term forms of psychotherapy or hospitalization, or who is willing to pool support services with other professionals will have a much greater chance of surviving.

- *Involvement in the general community*—The more widely known you are, the more opportunity you have to be a spokesperson for mental health issues and for yourself as an able practitioner. Participating in nonmedical community activities and being available to speak on mental health issues in the community are valuable means to this end.

Psychiatrists' Choices

Managed Care

Along with the general principles of practice building, real choices must be made. The first of these is planning to be in or out of the managed care system. This decision may be made by choice of specialty. Forensic psychiatry may be practiced independent of third-party oversight; geriatric psychiatry is heavily dependent on Medicare reimbursement, which involves fee restrictions, but not severe service limitations or concurrent review; and psychoanalytic practice must be conducted largely independently of the insurance system. These forms of practice may allow escape from the burdens and restrictions of third-party oversight, but may necessitate accepting reduced fees, having limited availability of work, and supplementing your practice with part-time salaried positions or other forms of practice.

Most practitioners must be involved in the managed care system to some significant degree, but can make choices about the extent of their participation and the type of plans in which to participate. An "all or nothing" attitude is likely to leave the psychiatrist disappointed and frustrated; a situation in which reimbursement comes in a variety of forms, including salary, third-party payment, and out-of-pocket payment may be the most satisfactory, especially in the earlier stages of one's career. This is not new to psychiatric practice. Surveys in the mid-1980s revealed that 70% of practicing psychiatrists worked in two or more settings and that more than one-half of psychiatric outpatients paid at least 50% of costs out-of-pocket, accounting for 25% of psychiatrists' gross incomes (Sharfstein and Beigel 1988). Thus, psychiatrists have been successfully operating in a mixed economy for some time.

To the extent that one works within the managed care system, it is important to recognize that all plans are not alike. Some clearly are interested in managing only cost, with little concern about the effect on care. Careful review of proposed contracts and consultation with other practicing psychiatrists will help the practitioner to detect such plans and avoid them as much as possible.

In dealing with the managed care programs you have selected, or with those that are unavoidable, it is important to adopt an attitude of collaboration, rather than contention. Such an attitude includes learning to speak to reviewers in a language they can understand about the need for and goals of treatment (Goodman et al. 1992). There is evidence that pressure from consumers of care (including businesses that contract for mental health benefits) and from legal liability are working against the survival of narrowly cost-motivated plans. Other plans, which aim for true cost-effectiveness and not merely cost control, may serve to stimulate genuine advances in the efficiency and efficacy of psychiatric treatment. Practitioners who are open-minded about attempting less costly treatments and skilled in talking to reviewers about additional needs of their patients will have the most credibility with ethical managed care companies.

Solo Versus Group Practice

Whether to practice alone or in a group is another important choice for beginning psychiatrists. It is still possible to conduct a "bare bones" solo office practice without clerical help, but it is increasingly difficult to do so. Computer software for billing and record keeping may help, but a major requisite for such a practice is having a base of patients who pay you directly, reliably, and with little or no associated paperwork. In the absence of such a base of patients (who are increasingly difficult to find), it may be necessary to take advantage of the economies of scale that come with some form of group affiliation. Such affiliations range from tightly knit partnerships, with coordinated clinical activities, to loose associations of practitioners who agree to share the expenses of offices and clerical help. In addition to administrative support, group affiliations may decrease professional isolation and increase referrals, although they come at a price of having to accommodate some of the needs of other professionals.

Practice Location

Another major choice is the type of practice location. Urban areas have historically been the most attractive practice locations for psychiatrists, but they may be glutted with mental health practitioners, both medical and nonmedical. In contrast, it is still common for psychiatrists practicing in smaller towns and rural areas to have more patient referrals than they can handle. To date, penetration of nonurban areas by managed care is less than in cities, and the practitioner is more likely to be able to develop a personal, collaborative relationship with reviewers. Thus, it may be substantially easier to build and maintain your chosen type of practice away from a major urban center. Such considerations must be weighed against the cultural and professional stimulation available in big cities.

The Future of Psychiatric Practice

What does the future hold for psychiatric practice? Certain trends seem clear. Long-term individual psychotherapy and long-term inpatient hospitalization will no longer be the core of the great majority of psychiatric practices. Instead, they will be replaced by a mixture of brief hospitalization, brief (or intermittent) psychotherapy, and psychopharmacological treatment. The core of psychiatric practice is undoubtedly shifting, but the range will continue to include some admixture of older forms of treatment in many practices and a predominance of them in some. Psychiatrists will spend more time in group practices and salaried work and less in solo private practice, although some amount of such work may continue to be essential for the morale of many practitioners. More, and probably most, of the care given by psychiatrists will be subject to third-party oversight of some type. As more outcome studies are performed, such oversight is likely to require explicit justification for any treatment without demonstrated efficacy. Medically and psychiatrically sicker patients will constitute a higher proportion of psychiatrists' caseloads than in recent decades. Elderly and seriously mentally ill patients are both increasing numerically in the population, and both have been historically underrepresented among private psychiatrists' patients (Goldman and Ridgely 1989). Population shifts and uneven geographical distribution of practitioners will pull greater numbers of psychiatrists away from northeastern "rust belt" urban centers into less populous regions of the Midwest, South, and Southwest.

What could cause the end to private psychiatric practice as we know it? One worst-case scenario would be for the federal government to prohibit physicians participating in a national health care system from contracting individually with patients for noncovered services. Because it would be very difficult for a psychiatrist to maintain a practice entirely outside a national system, such a regulation would drastically regiment and limit all but a few private practices. Furthermore, the internal rules of health collaboratives under national health care could limit the role of the psychiatrist to a high volume of brief patient contacts.

Short of limitation by the federal government, the greatest danger to psychiatric practice lies in domination of the field by managed care organizations that aim solely to reduce the cost of treatment. Under such circumstances, it would be impossible to develop a practice in the traditional way, based on a core of health professionals and patients who know you and the quality of your work. Instead, higher-priced care providers (including not only psychiatrists, but experienced and well-respected psychologists and social workers) would be largely excluded from the system in favor of those with minimal training and experience who would be willing to work at lower rates. Within such a system, the psychiatrist would not only work for less compensation, but would be barred from delivering any treatment except medication and electroconvulsive therapy. For many, if not most, psychiatrists, this would be an unacceptably narrow range of practice.

A third nightmare vision of future practice would be a system in which treatment was essentially dictated by managed care reviewers, with little room allowed for the physician's judgment. One occasionally hears stories about reviewers telling the psychiatrist what medication to prescribe, or insisting on sitting in on therapy sessions to judge the quality and necessity of treatment.

How likely are these outcomes? Prohibition of independent contracting by physicians is not part of currently proposed national health care legislation, but it could be written in later or imposed through regulation. Such regulations would be vehemently opposed by organized psychiatry and very likely by psychologists' organizations as well. Given the American value of freedom of choice, it is likely that the public would not readily accept a prohibition on purchasing affordable mental health services beyond those covered by the basic plan. There are also indications that harshly restrictive, cost-oriented managed care companies will not be allowed to take over the field. Vigilance by organized psychiatry and patient advocacy groups, as well as the dawn of legal liability for the outcome of managed care decisions, mitigate against wholesale abandonment of quality standards.

A recent outcome study (Rogers et al. 1993) indicated superiority of traditional fee-for-service over prepaid treatment for depressed outpatients. Future studies of this type may further clarify areas where traditional practice modes are advantageous and provide grounds for retaining them within the health care system.

Conclusion

Although we cannot be certain about the future, private practice of psychiatry remains alive and well in the present. Although most psychiatrists cannot practice just as they did 20 years ago, they are still able to adapt to changes without relinquishing their professional goals or compromising their integrity. Competence, energy, and flexibility remain the keys to success in private practice now, as they have in the past.

References

Anonymous: Adult psychiatry, private practice continue to be top choices among psychiatry residents. Psychiatric News, Volume 28, Number 11, June 4, 1993

Born DO: Psychiatric residents headed toward urban areas, private practice. Reece Report, Volume 7, Number 2, 1992, pp 5–15

Goldman HH, Ridgely MS: The future environment for psychiatry, in Future Directions for Psychiatry. Edited by Talbott JA. Washington, DC, American Psychiatric Association, 1989, pp 15–74

Goodman M, Brown J, Deitz P: Managing Managed Care. A Mental Health Practitioner's Survival Guide. Washington, DC, American Psychiatric Press, 1992

Rogers WH, Wells KB, Meredieth LS, et al: Outcomes for adult outpatients with depression under prepaid or fee-for-service financing. Arch Gen Psychiatry 50:517–525, 1993

Sharfstein S, Beigel A: How to survive in the private practice of psychiatry. Am J Psychiatry 145:700–707, 1988

Index

*Page numbers printed in **boldface** type refer to tables or figures.*